—— Putting ——
the Pieces Together

A Mother's Journey

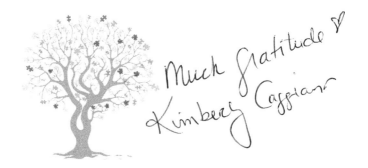

Much gratitude & Kimberly Caggiano

Our Story of an Autism Diagnosis

Kimberly M. Caggiano

PUTTING THE PIECES TOGETHER

ISBN: 978-0-578-70891-1

Design by Transcendent Publishing

Disclaimer: This book is not intended to diagnose, treat, cure, or prevent any disease and is not intended to be the medical advice of a physician. The reader should regularly consult a physician in matters relating to health and particularly with respect to any symptoms that may require diagnosis or medical attention.

Printed in the United States of America.

This is dedicated to Dylan, the little boy who has grown to be an amazing teenager and has accomplished what many said he would not.

I love you,

Mom

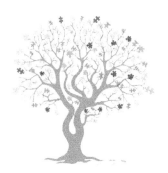

Your Special Needs Journey
has given you the stamina to
stand tall and face the
strongest of winds, your
branches full of faith and hope.
You were given this life because YOU
are strong enough to live it.

—A Very Special Needs Resource

Contents

Foreword

by
Anthony Caggiano

I want to start out by saying how honored and privileged I am to have the opportunity to write the foreword for this book, which has been a labor of love and devotion more than twelve years in the making.

I don't remember the exact day we knew, only that it all seemed to happen so fast. One moment our little boy was a fun, happy baby and the next he was being evaluated by doctors because he was not typically developing. I thought all toddlers had temper tantrums. I thought they all cried uncontrollably. I never would have known, if not for the keen intuition of my wife Kim, that he needed help. It is because of her that Dylan has had the best services, love and attention possible, because of her that he's had the opportunities to learn and develop in the way *his* brain is accustomed to. It is because of her that he has overcome seemingly insurmountable challenges to become the independent, smart and social young man he is today.

I recall like it was yesterday the night the idea for this book was birthed. It was about a year after Dylan's diagnosis, and Kim and I were talking about how much we had learned about Autism Spectrum Disorder in such a short period of time. We talked for hours about the progress he was making and renewed our commitment to provide him with the best options available. I commended her for the hard work she was doing with research and making sure that the path we took was going to benefit him over the long term.

"He is making great progress and learning every day," I told her. "He is the luckiest little boy in the world to have a mom like you, so dedicated and making it your mission to give him the right tools to learn."

Kim expressed gratitude for the services Dylan was receiving and said she wanted to share her knowledge and experiences with others facing similar challenges. She wanted them to know they were not alone, and possibly help them avoid the overwhelming helplessness we felt in the beginning. It was a great idea, but since being a mom to two sons, one of whom was on the spectrum, didn't leave her much time to write, that was pretty much where it ended. Over the next twelve years she would mention it every now and again, but life always seemed to get in the way.

During those years, Kim dedicated her entire life to our sons as a stay-at-home mom. She took this on without hesitation, tirelessly providing them not only with love and affection but discipline and hard lessons. Along the way she had gained enough knowledge to earn several PhDs in parenting and caring for a special needs child. Truly, the amount of reading, studying and advocacy she has done to make sure our son has received the services he needed is unfathomable.

Though I witnessed her efforts on a daily basis, they never failed to amaze me. I owned an IT consulting firm, and in the days before smart phones I used to have to run home between client appointments to check emails from the office in our spare bedroom. Each time I popped into the playroom to say hello I would find Kim playing or doing some kind of activity with Dylan. She would share with me what she had read the night before and what she was trying that day to get Dylan to talk or respond in certain ways. Day in and day out, whenever the PT, OT, SLP and ABA therapists were not there, Kim was, always trying to learn more, find out what worked for Dylan and understand how he learned best. She was not only helping our son move mountains, she was building the foundation so that as an adult he could live out his dreams and make his mark on the world.

Today, Dylan still struggles with some social interactions, but with the help and guidance of his mother and myself, he has made great strides. It has definitely not been easy, and I know there are many more challenges ahead as he continues to mature; however, I rest assured in the knowledge that we will face them together as a family.

As both our sons became more independent, Kim finally found the time needed to make the dream of writing this book a reality. It is as she envisioned it all those years ago – a learning guide for parents with a child newly diagnosed on the spectrum. It contains stories of the struggles we faced and the solutions that worked for us; it also goes into detail about different therapies and activities that she tried and the outcomes we experienced. But most of all, it is a book written from the heart, helping other parents who are feeling the emotions and daily struggles that come with raising a child on the spectrum, not with disabilities but with "different-abilities."

I hope you enjoy reading this book as much as I have and that it brings you the sense of comfort it was intended to bring. With that, I would like to welcome you to *A Mother's Journey*, written by one very dedicated, loving mother –my amazing wife, Kimberly Caggiano.

—Anthony Caggiano

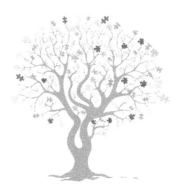

A Warm Welcome from the Author ...

Over the years, parents have regularly reached out to me for advice after their child was diagnosed with autism, and I was always immediately able to understand what they were going through. I vividly recall how my husband Anthony and I felt when our son Dylan was diagnosed at twenty-two months – panicked, terrified and shocked. Our plans for our life had just been upended, and we were unsure of where to turn or what to do. We just knew we had to find a new way forward. For me, that meant learning as much as I could about autism, including information that at the time was considered "cutting edge" or "pushing the envelope," depending on one's viewpoint. For the next twelve years I gathered that information, eventually ending up with multiple, well-organized binders. This book is the compilation of that research, along with the day-to-day struggles and victories we experienced as a family. It also contains support, tips and strategies, many of which came from the amazing professionals who worked with our family over the years. My appreciation for their expertise and their dedication to Dylan knows no bounds. All is designed to empower you to help your child realize his or her fullest potential.

I have also included assessments, test results and documentation for you to review if you haven't started the diagnosis yet. (For privacy purposes, all last names have been deleted from the documents from therapy sessions and appointments.) Consider documenting your story by utilizing the note sections created at the end of each chapter.

I must make it clear that I'm not a (professional) special education teacher, advocate or therapist, and my husband and I certainly don't have all the answers. What we have always had, however, is *hope,* and that, coupled with a lot of love and hard work, has paid off one hundredfold. Now fourteen, Dylan is doing amazing things that we were once told would never be within his reach. I pray that as you read along you feel empowered and know that you are part of a community. You are not alone. I also encourage you to find gratitude and joy in your journey, for this will become your pillar of strength in the days to come.

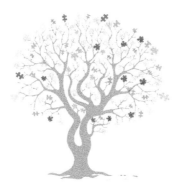

What is Early Intervention?

The impact that Early Intervention (EI) can have on a child's ability to learn new skills and overcome challenges cannot be overstated. EI is a system of publicly funded services that helps babies and toddlers with developmental delays or disabilities. Programs are available in every state and free for any child who is eligible; a doctor's referral is not necessary. Early intervention focuses on helping these children learn the skills that typically develop during the first three years of life, such as:

- **physical** (reaching, rolling, crawling, and walking)
- **cognitive** (thinking, learning, and solving problems)
- **communication** (talking, listening, and understanding)
- **social/emotional** (playing, feeling secure and happy)
- **self-help** (eating, dressing)

Who is on an Early Intervention Team?

Each EI team is a unique combination of professionals and laypersons, working together to help your child learn and overcome challenges. A Service Coordinator oversees the efforts of social-emotional specialists, behavioral specialists, assistive technology specialists, medical specialists, and childcare providers, all of whom bring knowledge and skills from their respective fields to the table. The most important team members, however, are your child and your family, including extended family members.

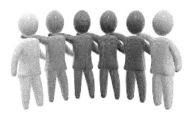

Family

- Knowledge about their family's culture in everyday routines
- Knowledge about their child and their family's needs

Service Coordinator

- Knowledge of the EI system
- Organizes the team
- Supports families through intake, evaluation, and Individual Family Service Plan (IFSP) process as well as the transition out of EI

Developmental Therapist

- Knowledge about child development and learning
- Helps families find ways to promote their child's development and learning through everyday routines and play
- Helps families understand how the IFSP goals fit together to promote overall child development

Occupational Therapist

- Knowledge of motor, self-help, and sensory development
- Helps families adapt every day activities based on their child's needs
- Focuses on fine motor skills such as feeding and grasping that require small muscles

Physical Therapist

- Knowledge of motor development and movement
- Helps families adapt every day activities based on their child's needs
- Focuses on gross motor skills such as crawling and walking that require large muscles

Speech and Language Pathologist

- Knowledge of language, feeding, and swallowing
- Helps families promote their child's language and communication development

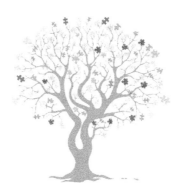

What is Autism Spectrum Disorder?

"If you've met one person with autism,
you've met one person with autism."

—Stephen Shore

There is no one type of autism, but many.

Autism encompasses a broad range of conditions characterized by challenges with social skills, repetitive behaviors, speech and nonverbal communication.

In 2013, the American Psychiatric Association merged four of these conditions – autistic disorder, childhood disintegrative disorder, pervasive developmental disorder-not otherwise specified (PDD-NOS), and Asperger syndrome – under the umbrella of autism spectrum disorder (ASD)[1]. There are also many subtypes of ASD, most of which are influenced

[1] Autismspeaks.org

by a combination of genetic and environmental factors. Because of this, each person with autism has a distinct set of strengths and challenges; moreover, the ways in which people with autism learn, think and problem-solve range from highly skilled to severely challenged. Some people with ASD may require significant support in their daily lives, while others may need less support and, in some cases, live entirely independently. According to the Centers for Disease Control, autism affects an estimated 1 in 59 children in the United States today.

Autism is often accompanied by sensory sensitivities and medical issues such as gastrointestinal (GI) disorders and seizures or sleep disorders, as well as mental health challenges such as anxiety, depression and attention issues. Indicators usually appear by age two or three, though some associated developmental delays can appear even earlier; oftentimes, it can be diagnosed as early as eighteen months. Research shows that, for people with autism, Early Intervention leads to positive outcomes later in life.

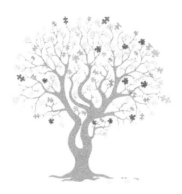

Timeline of Our Journey

May 5, 2008   Referral to Early Intervention

May 8, 2008   Early Intervention Assessment completed at initial home visit

July 8, 2008   Provisional Diagnosis by pediatrician

October 22, 2008   Evaluation at the National Autism Center

November 4, 2008   Official Diagnosis of Autistic Disorder

(DSM-IV 299.00)

August 31, 2009   Clinical Diagnostic Interview for Re-Evaluation at the National Autism Center. Re-Evaluation of current level of cognitive, social, emotional, and adaptive functioning. Previously seen at the clinic for comprehensive diagnostic evaluation on October 22, 2008.

October 6, 2009   Neurodevelopmental   Evaluation, including administration, scoring and interpreting the following psychological tests: Mullen Scales of Early Learning; Vineland Adaptive Behavior Scales (VABS); Child Behavior Checklist- parent form (CBCL); and the Autistic Diagnostic Observation Schedule, Module 2 (ADOS).

October 21, 2009 Parents received comprehensive feedback

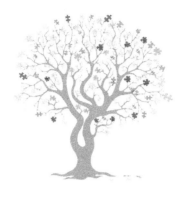

1

Evaluation and Assessment

"Autism is part of my child.
It's not everything he is.
My child is so much more than a diagnosis."

—S.L. Coelho

The Beginning Signs

Our journey began fourteen years ago, with the subtlest of signs. As I write this, I can't help but think back to those early days, when I would sit in the glider chair to feed Dylan and watch as he tapped his head and with his sweet little finger made circular motions on his forehead. Other times, he would be fascinated by the blades of the ceiling fan as they went round and round. Friends and family would often remark, "What a quiet baby he is!"

For a few months we met with the pediatrician and voiced our concerns, but each time he explained that it was common for baby boys to exhibit this type of behavior. He also told us that Dylan was too young to test. Anthony and I had little choice but to believe him. We were new parents, facing the typical learning curve, and since our friends didn't have children yet we had nothing to compare our experience with. Besides, Dylan was such an easy baby; he smiled often and was easily calmed.

At around twelve months, the signs became more obvious. He was frustrated with limited verbal and nonverbal communication and would have intense tantrums and start hitting and banging his head wherever he could. It started happening every day, multiple times a day.

To say this was a difficult time would be a gross understatement. It became harder and harder to convince ourselves that this was typical behavior for two-year-olds, though not for lack of trying. One day I was talking to my sweet mother-in-law Rosanne, a retired kindergarten teacher with over forty years of experience. Her knowledge and love of children was something I had always admired and respected. She suggested we contact the local Early Intervention for a free evaluation.

"Even if nothing comes up," she said, "we'll at least have that peace of mind."

Prior to her mentioning it, I wasn't familiar with Early Intervention, or frankly I would've called much sooner. Still, I dreaded the thought of it. I vividly remember the day, May 5, 2008, when as Dylan lay napping I picked up the phone and dialed the number my mother-in-law had found for me.

"What specifically are your concerns?" asked the woman on the other end of the line.

I told her that Dylan was very aggressive and that his tantrums and meltdowns were so intense that he was hurting himself. As we spoke, my heart was racing, along with my thoughts. Whatever happened with Early Intervention, I knew there would be no turning back, no more telling ourselves that Dylan was typically developing.

The Evaluation

The initial home visit evaluation took place just a few days later, on May 8th. Evaluators from multiple disciplines – Occupational Therapy, Physical Therapy, and Speech and Language Therapy – as well as an Early Intervention Specialist and a Case Manager came to our home, the goal being to observe and interact with Dylan at the same time and begin compiling a collaborative and comprehensive evaluation of his strengths and challenges. The EI team looked at the following six functional areas of development:

Fine motor/perceptual – How he coordinated his eyes and hands to reach, grasp, and handle objects

Language – How he communicated and understood what people said to them

Cognition – How he solved problems, imitated and played

Social/emotional – How he interacted with others and his environment

Gross motor – How he coordinated the large muscles of his body to move

Self-help/adaptive – How he was developing with regard to feeding, toileting and dressing skills

My husband, mother-in-law and I were not prepared for such a crowd and unsure what to expect. I was overwhelmed with worry and more than a little emotional, but I managed to pull myself together, put on my social worker hat, and observe as each discipline spent time evaluating him on the floor of our living room.

When the evaluation was complete we moved into the kitchen and stood around the island as each took turns talking to us about their findings. I'll never forget the insensitive, almost flippant demeanor of one woman as she said, "Dylan definitely showed signs of autism, but we're not doctors, so we can't diagnose."

The three of us exchanged looks of confusion and disbelief. Autism? No way. Of course I had heard of it, I knew there were families "out there" dealing with it, but what did "signs of autism" mean for Dylan? I just kept thinking, *He has a speech issue... that's all,* yet at the same time I felt as though my world had stopped. One look at Anthony told me his had as well. Shocked, upset and unsure what to say or do, I respectfully but firmly asked the team to leave immediately.

Twenty-four hours later, I called Early Intervention back. After giving it much thought and talking to my husband, friends, family, and mother-in-law, I had decided I wouldn't let one unprofessional team member rob Dylan or us of the help we needed. I explained to EI how upsetting her comment and demeanor was and requested that she not return. Remember, the team of therapists who initially comes to your home must provide information that is clear, specific, and understandable. Just as importantly, they must do so with the highest sensitivity. This type of visit is stressful enough.

Have you ever heard the saying, "Sometimes things have to fall apart in order for them to fall back together?" Well, that's what happened here. The EI team came back the next day, minus the insensitive woman but with the sweetest and knowledgeable case manager we ever could've asked for. From the moment she entered our home Karen was like a shining star – kind, compassionate, a great listener, and she answered all of our questions patiently. We instantly knew we were in good hands.

This time, after the team had assessed Dylan, we were given a written summary, in which the team member from each of the disciplines had documented their findings. It explained the age level at which Dylan had scored and recommended the appropriate services. The Service Coordinator reviewed the assessment with us and explained how each service would be provided. Below, you will find Dylan's assessment so you have a reference for what one should look like.

Name: _____ Age: 27 mos. Date of Evaluation: 5/8/08

This summary of your child's assessment will be followed by a more complete report that your service coordinator will review with you.

Cognition	Age level	Recommendations:
[handwritten] Matched 2 select items Identified objects by use Slow to imitate	23 mos.	*[handwritten]* encourage imitation of actions, gestures and movement
Language	Age level Expressive: Receptive:	Recommendations:
Processes auditory information well. Follows novel directions well. Uses well over +50 single words. Beginning to use simple 2 word phrases	23 months	- Appears to be excellent progress over the past month - Playgroup would be great! *[handwritten]* judgement for evaluation
Gross Motor	Age level	Recommendations:
Starting to walk down stairs with hand held. Attempts to jump. Squats in play. Climbs onto adult furniture	17 months	Stepping up and down curb height with hand held.
Fine Motor	Age level	Recommendations:
Did complete a 3 piece formboard. Stacked 3 blocks. Imitated some vertical and horizontal stroking with crayon in fisted grasp	22 months	Writing on easel
Social/Emotional	Age level	Recommendations:
happy, lively, busy. *[handwritten]* eye contact can be expressive *[handwritten]* has difficulty with transition	27 mos.	Play group!
Self Care	Age level	Recommendations:
[handwritten] with toothbrush & vibration. Continues *[handwritten]* Uses utensils. Begin *[handwritten]* toilet train	Dressing 22 Feeding 31 Toileting 26	- Oral motor evaluation for low oral sensitivity - Try the "p"

(Early Intervention Summary of Assessment, 2008)

May 8, 2008 27 months

Summary of Child's Assessment

Cognition: 23 months

Good attention and enthusiasm

Matched 2 sets of items

Identified objects by use

Slow to imitate

Recommendations: encourage imitation of actions, gestures, and movement

Language: 23 months

Processes auditory information well

Follows novel directions well

Uses well over +/- 50 single words

Beginning to use simple 2-word phrases

Recommendations: Appears to be excellent progress over the past month, playgroup should be considered, clinical judgement for frustration

Gross Motor: 17 months

Starting to walk down the stairs with hand held

Attempts to jump

Squats in play

Climbs onto adult furniture

Recommendations: Stepping up and down curb height with hand held

Fine Motor: 22 months

Did complete a 3-piece form board

Stacked 3 blocks

Initiated vertical and horizontal stroking with crayon in fisted grasp

Recommendations: Writing on an easel

Social/Emotional: 27 months

Happy, lively boy

Can be aggressive when frustrated

Difficulty with transition

Recommendation: Play group

Self-Care (Dressing 22 months low due to clothing sensitivity; Feeding 31 months; Toileting 26 months)

Cooperates with tooth brushing with vibration

Continues to mouth non-edibles

Uses utensils

Beginning to toilet train

<u>Recommendations:</u> Oral Motor Evaluation for low oral sensitivity

(Detailed Summary of Assessment)

Parent Tip: During the evaluation the EI staff will decide if your child's behavior during the assessment is typical. The staff may ask you additional questions about how your child usually interacts with people and situations and while playing with their toys. There will be an opportunity for you to ask questions. They may offer suggestions and provide their overall impression of your child. After having a conversation with you, and gathering information obtained from the multidisciplinary assessment and observation of your child, they will discuss the initial eligibility evaluation. This will include information as to whether your child's skill development and behavior is typical of other children of that age. This indicates if there is a delay found in one or more areas of development. This information is a written description of the assessment/evaluation called Developmental Profile. Based upon the information gathered during the initial evaluation/assessment process, your child may or may not be eligible for EI services.

Below is Dylan's completed Developmental Profile. As you will see, the Profile summarizes the assessment/evaluation gathered regarding his health and development, including

Social Emotional/Interaction, Cognition, Gross Motor, Fine Motor, Communication and Self-Care.

Social Emotional/Interaction: 27 months
- Lively, friendly and sociable boy
- Good eye contact
- Loves to play outside
- High activity level
- Has some difficulty with transitions-can become very upset
- Can be aggressive with peers in social situations, and is often aggressive with caregivers
- Limited opportunities to interact with peers-playgroup is recommended

Cognition: 23 months
- Good attention to activities while seated in a high chair
- Matched 2 sets of items
- Identified objects by use
- Not readily imitative of actions, gestures and movements

Gross Motor: 17 months
- Walks with control
- Takes steps sideways
- Able to take a few steps backwards with encouragement
- Able to walk up some stairs with two hands on railing
- Crawls up stairs
- Climbs onto adult furniture
- Stepping up and down low curb height with minimal assistance
- Equilibrium reaction in sit and stand appear delayed
- Attempts to jump in place

Fine Motor: 22 months
- Used two hands together to attempt to fold paper, turn pages of cardboard book and remove cover from a small box
- Completed reversed formboard
- Stacked 3 cubs
- Imitated aligning cubes to form a train
- Tendency to fist crayon
- Imitated some vertical and horizontal scribbling
- Required assistance to unscrew a jar lid

Communication: Receptive: 23 months   Expressive: 23 months
- Very outgoing and social with new evaluators
- Processes auditory information quickly and accurately
- Follows new directions immediately
- Easily identified pictures, objects and body parts
- Understands the function of objects
- Reportedly is using well over 50 single words to label and answer questions
- Beginning to show physical signs of frustration
- Emerging 2-3 word sentences by report

- Clarity of speech is age appropriate for single words
- Demonstrates signs and symptoms of low oral sensitivity
- Frequently mouths non edibles
- Hearing tested at birth and reported as normal

Self-Care:
Feeding: 31 months
- Likes a variety of food and textures (loves cold temps)
- Recently pacifier use has decreased
- Uses utensils independently
- Craves oral deep pressure

Toileting: 26 months
- Beginning to toilet train
- Uses words to indicate the need to use the bathroom

Dressing/Hygiene: 22 months
- Attempts to brush his hair but reportedly is sensitive to hats or things on his head
- Does not cooperate with face or hand washing
- Now likes to have his teeth brushed with a vibrating toothbrush

(Developmental Profile, 2008)

Parent Tip: If your child is found to be eligible for EI services, a member from the team will work with you to develop an Individualized Family Service Plan, also called an IFSP. The IFSP will delineate outcomes or goals that may be achieved in a number of ways. It may include activities, services, treatment or intervention options necessary to support your child's development. They will assist you in finding resources and support to help you care for your child. An IFSP is a flexible plan that changes as the child grows and develops. It must be rewritten every year and reviewed at least once every six months. Specific outcomes and strategies, as well as the names and professional disciplines of service providers, are defined in the IFSP.

According to Dylan's full Assessment/Developmental Profile, he was experiencing a delay in gross motor skills, fine motor skills, and speech and language; he also scored significantly low on cognition, social/emotional interactions, had difficulty with transitions (switching from one activity to another) and could be aggressive with both peers and caregivers. As such, he was determined eligible for Early Intervention Services, which begins with the creation of the Individualized Family Services Plan, of IFSP.

Early intervention services must be individualized according to the strengths, needs, and resources of the particular child and their family. The IFSP is the basis for all services and support tools. As noted in the box above, this comprehensive plan includes information about your family's strengths, needs and routines. An IFSP will also include written outcomes, or goals, that the family hopes their child will attain. Parents and EI staff work together to determine these outcomes and in deciding what approaches will be used to reach them. Of course, a parent can always decline services. On the other hand, if the team finds that your child is not eligible for EI services, they will most likely make every effort to help you identify other ways to support your child's growth and development through other home- or community-based resources and activities.

Karen, our Developmental Specialist, reviewed and explained thoroughly what the Service Delivery Plan is, how it works and, if necessary, how it could be modified. For us, services would be provided Monday through Friday and were as follows:

Home visit 1xw (once per week) to guide and discuss progress with a Developmental Specialist
Physical therapy 2xw
Occupational therapy 2xw
Speech and language therapy 2xw
Playgroup 2xw, one-on-one in a structured environment while parents wait.
(Behavioral Therapy would be added *after* a formal diagnosis was provided.)

Below are Dylan's Desired Family Outcomes and Strategies created by the Service Coordinator in collaboration with me and Anthony.

Outcomes:

1. He will be able to communicate better and have less frustration.
2. He will use his words to identify his wants and needs and be less frustrated when people don't understand him.
3. He will use words instead of biting, hitting, banging his head to express emotions.
4. He will have an easier time with transitions.
5. Dylan will have social time with his peers.
6. He will learn to use words to communicate and not use aggressive behaviors. He will learn to be more comfortable transitioning from one activity to another.

Strategies:

1. When you know what he wants, give him the words. If he points to juice, say, "Juice. You want juice? Here's your juice." Use an excited voice and do a lot of repetition. Narrate his play, again with lots of repetition and using mostly one or two words at a time. Name actions as well as nouns.

2. Give him the words for his emotions (i.e. "You're mad"/"I'm mad").

3. Give him choices. "Do you want juice or milk?"; "Do you want to do up or down?"; "Do you want to wear the red or blue shirt?"

4. Give him two or three heads up before transitions. Create Social Stories.

5. Attend weekly playgroups so he learns to co-operate with transitions and routines.

(Desired Family Outcomes and Strategies, 2008)

From the moment that plan was put into action, my daily routine took an abrupt and dramatic turn. As Anthony worked very long days, I was responsible for Dylan's treatment. Each morning a different therapist from Early Intervention showed up at our home, followed by additional therapists throughout the day. They would see us at our best and our worst. I always tried to make sure we were up and ready to begin so Dylan received the most out of each service, even if that meant we were still in our pajamas.

It wasn't easy. The days seemed endless, and I was emotionally and physically exhausted from Dylan's biting, hitting and frustration. I was also drowning in paperwork as I tried to keep up with his schedule (which therapists were coming each day), as well the new jargon, information and suggestions that were continually pouring in. I mean, there were papers *everywhere.* I knew if I wanted to stay sane and grounded, I had to find a way to simplify everything that I possibly could. Before I knew it I had compiled everything into several three-ring binders. I also created a form called the **Early Intervention Home Schedule,** which allowed me to organize my own notes as well as the notes the therapists provided me on each visit.

I printed enough copies of the Schedule for weeks at a time and attached them to a clipboard that I placed next to the binders on the kitchen counter. At the end of each week, I'd simply add the sheets to the binder. Below is an example of that form. *(Please visit www.PuttingThePiecesTogetherBook. com to print free copies.)*

EI would continue for the next few months. Though each therapist (OT, PT, SLA, Service Coordinator) had their own methods and goals for working with Dylan, they all arrived for their sessions with a bin or large bag filled to the brim with toys. Dylan would stand in front of the window, jumping up and down with excitement to see what they had with them that day. I would gather my clipboard and observe from a distance so I wasn't distracting to him, and I was always impressed by the therapists' professionalism and kindness as they engaged with Dylan.

I also remember listening intently, trying to write down any catch phrases or new terminology that was unfamiliar. I felt it was imperative to be consistent with what they were doing in order to see the best results moving forward.

Early Intervention Home Schedule

Today's Date: _____

Today's Schedule:

Occupational Therapy _____   Specialty MD Appt _____

Physical Therapy _____   Pediatrician _____

Behavioral Therapy _____   Play Group _____

Speech and Language Therapy _____

Notes/Observation:

_____
_____
_____
_____
_____
_____
_____
_____
_____
_____
_____
_____
_____
_____
_____
_____
_____

Questions:

_____
_____
_____
_____
_____
_____

Upcoming Appointments and Questions to Ask:

_____
_____
_____
_____

During the session, I would come up with symbols to correspond with my notes so I could easily review them that night or teach them to Anthony over the weekend. For example, an asterisk (*) meant to ask about what was being taught, and an exclamation mark (!) meant Anthony and I needed to learn certain phrases/words.

I soon found myself giving one hundred percent of every day to Dylan's services, and though it was a lot of work with a steep learning curve it also felt very natural to me. Before becoming a wife and mother I had worked in the Social Work field, specifically in case management, therapeutic recreation, geriatrics, and as Director of an Alzheimer's Unit in an Assisted Living facility. I was used to, and thoroughly enjoyed, advocating for others, and I truly believed (and still do) that God sent me Dylan so I could utilize those skills to the best of my knowledge and ability.

That said, taking charge of my son's treatment was much more emotionally and physically challenging than caring for clients. There were times when I felt trapped in the house and very isolated, as we had moved to a new town shortly before Dylan's diagnosis and didn't know many people. I looked forward to seeing the smiling faces of the Early Interventions' staff that came to our house each morning. Some offered a hug on really hard days, which made me feel better and more confident about embarking on this new journey. Whenever I needed to feel supported in what I was doing, they were there.

The next step in the process was to choose a specialty service of Behavioral Therapy: Applied Behavioral Analysis (ABA) or Floortime (I will describe them both in detail later on); however, in order to do this we needed a "firm diagnosis" of autism. Karen suggested we find a new pediatrician, one who was familiar with autism and comfortable treating children on the spectrum. She provided us with the Early Intervention Development Profile; Parent Report; Clinical Observation

Report; and Social-Emotional Report to present to the doctor we chose. Now, in addition to my other tasks, I was consumed with researching and interviewing doctors. My mother-in-law was a godsend, watching Dylan while I went to one appointment after another. Though I was impressed with each of these physicians, my gut would tell me they weren't the one. I was looking for someone special; someone with whom I connected and would respect our plan in place. It took three weeks, but I found a gem of a pediatrician, Dr. Leslie. She was a mom of two young boys and had grown up with a brother on the autism spectrum. Perfect! It was such a relief to know we were headed in the right direction.

On July 8, 2008, Dr. Leslie thoroughly examined Dylan and provided a "Provisional Diagnosis of Autism Spectrum Disorder" based on a clinical assessment, review of his developmental evaluations, and the administration of the Modified

Date: 07/08/2008 12:27 PM

RE:
DOB:

To Whom It May Concern:

This patient is enrolled in an early intervention program. I have made a provisional diagnosis of autism spectrum disorder on this patient based on my clinical assessment, review of his developmental evaluations, and administration of the Modified Checklist for Autism in Toddlers (M-CHAT).
Please enroll this child in a Specialty Services early intervention program for children with autism spectrum disorders.

Sincerely,

Rererrals made:
_____ General EI (already enrolled in Westfield Infant Toddler)
___X_ Audiology

(Provisional Diagnosis from pediatrician)

Checklist for Autism in Toddlers (M-CHAT). The Provisional Diagnosis was sufficient for us to choose our specialty service, and we decided on ABA.

The next goal was to find a doctor or clinic to begin the "Official Diagnosis" process. Karen provided us with a packet of Diagnostic Evaluation Resources, which included three pages of doctors (names, addresses and phone numbers) in our area. I called each and every one only to hear about their long waiting list. I was starting to feel overwhelmed and worried. The days were going by and we needed a "firm diagnosis" to begin ABA. When I told Karen of my concerns, she asked if we'd consider traveling to the Boston area, where The May Institute National Autism Center was located. It wasn't even a question – Anthony and I would have gone anywhere to get the testing started. I called the Center and scheduled the initial appointment, a Parent Interview lasting approximately ninety minutes, for September 30, 2008.

Once again, my mother-in-law babysat for Dylan while we headed to the appointment. She was excited to have the day with her grandson and Anthony and I were happy to have uninterrupted alone time in the car. (We had almost forgotten what that had felt like!) As we pulled into the parking lot of the Center we were nervous but confident that we could provide an accurate description of where Dylan was on a day-to-day basis. He had made strides over the past months with EI, but the additional services he could get following an official diagnosis promised more growth. It was a powerful motivator.

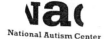

Autism Spectrum Disorders Assessment Clinic

An Outreach Clinic of May Institute

National Autism Center

September 17, 2008

Dear   ,

Enclosed are directions to the National Autism Center, as well as forms to be completed by parent(s) and school or caregiver professionals prior to your initial appointment. Please complete these forms and bring them with you to your appointment, along with any other records that you would like to share with your clinician.

As a reminder, your appointment is scheduled is **September 30th at 3:00 pm.** This is parent interview, and will take approximately 90 minutes.

Your child does not need to attend this appointment, and it is preferable that he/she is not present. However, we realize that this is not always possible. Therefore, if you need to bring any children to the appointment, you may, but please notify the office of this in advance. Unfortunately, we do not provide child care services.

If you need to cancel or reschedule your appointment for any reason, please notify   at least 24 hours in advance of your appointment. We look forward to seeing you.

Sincerely,

The Clinic Team
ASD Diagnostic Clinic
Autism Spectrum Disorders Assessment Clinic
National Autism Center

(May Center National Autism Center, letter initial appointment, 9/17/08)

As a result of that initial appointment, Dylan was scheduled for a Comprehensive Diagnostic Evaluation on October 22, 2008. He was then referred for a Neuro-Developmental Evaluation, which would assess his current cognitive, social, emotional and adaptive functioning.

That morning, we were welcomed by a warm receptionist and asked to take a seat in the lobby until we were called in.

We were fifteen minutes early – enough time to be anxious! – but the lobby was bright and sunny and Dylan was happy and doing well, which helped us relax a bit.

When it was time, we walked down a large, open beautiful hallway, looking at the photos on the wall of the events they held and the children who attended their programs. Suddenly, the emotions I had carefully held in check over the past months started bubbling to the surface. I had been going all day, non-stop, with no time for myself, our marriage or daily life to get to this point. As always, Anthony knew when I needed support and enveloped me in a hug. I instantly felt better, and knew that comforting me strengthened him as well.

We met the intern and doctor, who explained that we would be able to observe the evaluation from behind the glass that overlooked the testing room. Though I regularly watched Dylan with EI staff in our home and at EI play groups, I found this session especially interesting. Still, I didn't take as many notes that day, as I was too busy praying for the best possible outcome.

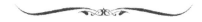

Journal your thoughts and feelings about the moment you heard the words, "Your child has autism," and how it has affected your family.

_____

_____

_____

_____

_____

_____

_____

_____

_____

_____

_____

_____

_____

_____

_____

_____

_____

_____

_____

_____

_____

_____

_____

_____

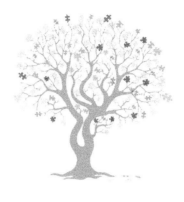

2

Diagnosis and Plan

"When people meet someone with autism, they all too often assume they understand that individual's challenges and strengths simply because of the diagnosis. That is not the case. As the saying goes, "If you've met one person with autism, you've met one person with autism."

—Kerry Magro

Diagnosis

Anthony and I sat across the desk from the doctor, staring down at the copy of the diagnosis report she had handed us. We had been waiting for this day for months; we had worked through our denial by educating ourselves and being resourceful. We were prepared for an official diagnosis – we had even advocated for it. Yet as she began to review her findings it felt very different than we had imagined. I thought back to what my Aunt Donna, who had been a special education teacher for thirty-eight years, had said to us the night before: "The diagnosis doesn't define him. He will still be the same boy you love and adore, and you will always be his parent first and his teacher second."

Now, I struggled to hold onto those wise words as the doctor gently stated that Dylan had met specific criteria for a

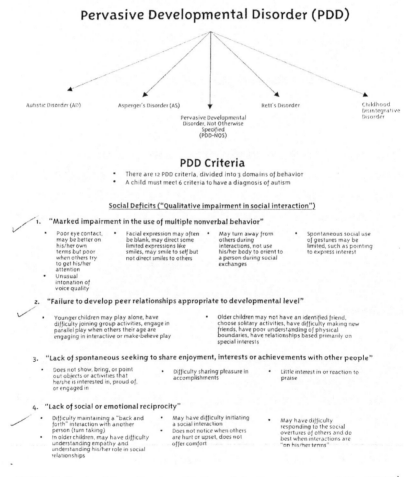

(PDD Criteria, May Center, National Autism Center, MA, 2008)

diagnosis of PDD-NOS/Autistic Disorder. Though I knew beyond a shadow of a doubt that my aunt had spoken the truth, it still felt like the world as we knew it was crumbling around us. The doctor handed us a box of tissues and we just cried and tried to process the enormity of the situation. And in that moment, the last bits of denial we had unknowingly been clinging to disappeared for good.

Communication Deficits ("Qualitative impairment in communication")

1. "Delay in, or total lack of, the development of spoken language"

   - Any significant early delay in language development (receptive and expressive)
   - There is no attempt to compensate for the delay with other ways of communicating, like gestures and mime

2. "Marked impairment in the ability to initiate or sustain a conversation"

   - This does not apply to children who do not have phrase language
   - May have one-sided exchanges, talk "at" you rather than with you, have trouble answering open-ended questions, trouble starting/stopping conversations, difficulty talking about topics not of special interest

3. "Stereotyped and repetitive use of language or idiosyncratic language"

   - Immediate echolalia
   - Jargon
   - Formal, pedantic style of speaking
   - Repeating lines from favorite videos, books
   - Scripted or "canned" use of phrases
   - Pronoun reversal (I/you)

4. "Lack of varied, spontaneous make-believe play or social imitative play"

   - Play that is not at a developmentally appropriate age
   - In young children, lack of interest in social games, such as peek-a-boo
   - In older children, lack of appropriate pretend play

Repetitive Behaviors ("Restricted, repetitive, and stereotyped patterns of behavior, interest or activities")

1. "Encompassing preoccupation with one or more stereotyped and restricted patterns of interest that is abnormal either in intensity or focus"

   - In younger children, may be an intense interest in certain videos, like *Thomas*, in certain toys, like trains or cars, in numbers and letters, in mechanical objects such as elevators, etc.
   - In older children, this might include intense interest in certain subjects that he/she knows many facts about, such as marine mammals, outer space, dinosaurs, etc
   - Excellent memory for details of special interests

2. "Apparently inflexible adherence to specific, nonfunctional routines or rituals"

   - Needing to do things in a particular manner, order, or sequence, and becoming distraught is that order is not followed
   - Examples: schedule routines, eating routines, placement routines (e.g., where furniture is located in the house), dressing routines

3. "Stereotyped and repetitive motor mannerisms"

   - Hand flapping
   - Finger flicking
   - Spinning
   - Body posturing (moving the body into unusual and repetitive postures)
   - Pacing
   - Running in circles
   - Rocking
   - Walking on tip toe

4. "Persistent preoccupations with parts of objects"

   - Interests that seem sensory in nature
   - Lining up or spinning objects
   - Repetitive dropping of objects, or watching objects fall (water, sand, balls, etc.)
   - Visual examination of parts of toys (e.g., the wheels on a car), squinting or peering

(PDD Criteria, May Center, National Autism Center, MA, 2008)

She proceeded to show us a diagram (above) that explained the findings, but my husband and I wanted more. What did this actually mean for Dylan? For his future, and for our family on a day- to-day basis?

It's been twelve years, and that day, that moment, remains frozen in my mind. I suspect it always will be. The feelings of sadness and loss were profound as she gently explained that Dylan would probably not potty train until at least the age of nine, never ride a bike or be able to handle riding a swing of any kind. He would need one-on-one care. Devastated doesn't begin to describe how we felt. We knew they had an obligation to provide us that information, but that didn't lessen the pain. Early Intervention had always made things hopeful for us; the way this was presented felt like our son had a label, and he did. Life was about to change again and I truly didn't know how I was going to face it. My husband, always a pillar of strength, really stepped up to the plate. He became strong when I was weak; he knew he needed to do that because if I fell apart, we all would.

Parent Tip: When you leave the meeting, allow yourself time to process what you have heard. Don't do anything or make any big decisions. If possible, schedule an appointment to go back another time or schedule a phone call to follow up. It may take a few days to process the initial shock. Prepare for the call with a paper/pen and questions about what the next steps should be. Everyone feels and processes a new diagnosis differently. Take time for yourself and partner; allow some grace during this stressful time.

After receiving Dylan's diagnosis, Anthony and I were handed the paperwork and sent on our way. We talked and cried the whole way home, but at the same time we felt a strange sense of relief. Now that we knew what was going on and were beginning to understand more about autism, we could help him. No parent is ever really prepared to hear that their child has ASD. Hearing those words brings on a rush of paralyzing worry; you're unsure of what to do next and confused by conflicting advice from multiple people trying to help point you in the right direction. Added to this is the fear that ASD may be an incurable condition, which keeps your focus on possible future struggles rather than where it needs to be: your child's needs in the present.

Parent Tip: If you are feeling confused and over-whelmed, it's because you have entered a territory that is unfamiliar to you. The solution to feeling empowered is to start educating yourself about ASD (i.e. the terminology). Knowledge is power, as they say and, over time you'll feel more in control because the knowledge you've gained helps you make informed decisions for your child. Be patient and kind to yourself.

Once the initial shock of the diagnosis begins to fade, many parents are left wondering, *Why my child? How did this happen?* I know we felt this way. We began to think, *I'm not sure we can do this. This is a lot.* I also felt a lot of anger around Dylan's diagnosis and was terrified about the challenges it would mean for him and our family moving forward. In the coming months I would often become angry that some of our family and friends didn't understand or want to understand, and that parents kept away from us at the park or avoided playdates with Dylan because he was biting, hitting or having a meltdown.

These emotions were both confusing and overwhelming for me because I had always been such a positive person. Now the usual uplifting words and thoughts I used to get me through the rough times were not working. Then I recalled the life lesson offered by one of my college professors years earlier: "When you become an adult, you're going to have very hard days. Don't stay in that place or dwell in that place; always give yourself twenty-four hours and move on. Find ways to work through the problem or issue to resolve it." I had always found this to be profound; now they became my words to live by. No amount of grieving or denial would change the diagnosis. What Dylan needed was for us to be focused and prepared, and remembering that would enable us to push through.

> **Parent Tip**: You have the right to feel angry, but be careful because unchecked or misdirected anger carries a lot of negative energy. Instead, try using your anger in a positive way by refocusing your direction. Also, take the time you need and process it by reaching out to a good friend or local support group or counselor.

We knew this, and still it was a constant battle. In fact, sometimes it was unbearable. I often felt hopeless and invisible, broken and isolated. Now, as I look back on those tough days, I realize I used those emotions to motivate, inspire and drive me to do more, learn more, and to be more for Dylan. I eventually became so tired of being angry that I would do anything I could to free myself. The key was acceptance. At the end of the day, we don't need to know it all, we just need to love and accept our children as they are, unconditionally. We need to fully accept the diagnosis and how life is now, and to begin to feel gratitude for the joy and the goodness in our lives. "G*row* through what you *go* through" needs to become our motto.

In the days and months following the diagnosis, Anthony and I took care of each other and resumed "normal" life as best we could while working through the fears, denial, distress, grief and panic. Dylan deserved the opportunity to learn and grow to the best of his capabilities, whatever that meant for him. It was a great comfort that we had one of the best Early Intervention teams in the county at our disposal and we felt confident with the process that lie ahead.

Parent Tip: Give your marriage extra TLC during this time. Find a trusted babysitter or ask a family member to help so you can go out; if this isn't an option you might sit together on the couch talking and connecting. Continue to make quality time for each other, keep the communication open and find moments to laugh, especially on the hard days.

There were many times, both after the diagnosis and for many years afterward, when I found myself drained emotionally. I felt depleted from fighting for everything and advocating for Dylan and our family, and some days all I could think about was how I'd make it through. My go-to reaction in those days was to push everyone away. Essentially, I had become a martyr. My husband and close friends have understood and continue to love me through it, while many others were never able to grasp what I was going through.

Like most parents, I suspect, Anthony and I have often joked that we wished there were an instruction manual or special class on raising children. There isn't, of course, and certainly not for parents of children with autism. During the early years, it seemed whenever when we thought we had a good handle on managing day-to-day issues and Dylan's behaviors, he would change and we'd have to figure out other alternatives. I still fight every

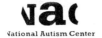

National Autism Center

Autism Spectrum Disorders Assessment Clinic
An Outreach Clinic of May Institute

November 4, 2008

Dear Mr. and Mrs

This letter is to confirm that we met today for a feedback appointment to discuss your son's evaluation that took place on October 22, 2008 at the National Autism Center's Autism Spectrum Disorder Assessment Clinic.

As discussed, I have diagnosed your son with Autistic Disorder (DSM-IV: 299.00). He meets seven of the twelve stated criteria at this time. I have recommended that Dylan receive at least 25 hours of service that includes Applied Behavior Analysis implemented by a certified ABA therapist, speech and language services, and occupational therapy for fine motor, sensory, and adaptive concerns. He would also continue to benefit from structured play groups. Dylan's program of services should be year round for maximum effectiveness. Services can be offered at home and/or at school once he turns 3.

If you have any further questions about your son's diagnosis or treatment plan, please feel free to contact me at   . I have enjoyed meeting Dylan and working with your family.

Sincerely,

(National Autism Center, MA, Official Diagnosis, 11/4/2008)

day, though the nature of the fight has changed as he has grown and evolved. With Anthony's strength and support, I've learned to take it one day at a time and sometimes one minute at a time.

The Plan

On November 4, 2008 we received the official diagnosis in the mail, along with other documentation the Early Intervention team needed to move forward with the Behavioral Therapy. As mentioned before, there were different options under this category, Floortime and Applied Behavioral Analysis (ABA). This intensive home-based therapy was tailored to meet each child's specific needs. We decided on ABA based on input from EI and the doctor who diagnosed Dylan, as well as what appeared to be most effective for his specific needs. Karen gave us pamphlets for three different agencies so I could begin the process of interviewing Specialty Providers.

Dylan became very frustrated when he couldn't communicate his feelings, thoughts, wants and needs, and oftentimes this manifested as aggression aimed at me in the form of hitting, kicking and biting me. Karen explained that this was because I was the closest person to him all day and loved him unconditionally. He knew that and felt he could trust me. Understanding the why didn't make it any easier to deal with. Some bites broke the skin and instantly bruised. When it was at its worst the therapists would wrap my arms and legs in ace bandages so I would have protection. Though he couldn't control his behavior, Dylan was apologetic for it, which he demonstrated with warm hugs. The therapists suggested I try not to respond or cry in front of him when the biting occurred, but after a while I started to just break down, not just because of the physical pain but the stress of daily appointments, tantrums and meltdowns.

I journaled a lot during this period, which helped me process my feelings. I also found out very quickly who was part of my support system and who wasn't. Anthony was my rock, and I relied on him heavily every day. As mentioned earlier, though, certain friends couldn't or wouldn't understand, while others were there only when I was having a particularly rough day. A few friends, as well as my mother-in-law and aunt, supported me every step of the way, and they still do. Even if your support system is one person, be sure to say what you need and how they can be helpful to you. Sometimes, it's just a matter of someone coming to play with your child for a half-hour so you can take a shower, or listening to you while you vent without judgement. Most importantly, you have to be your own support system. Find ways to nourish yourself, laugh and love. Laughter, daily affirmations and listening to music have always been healing for me.

Use daily affirmations to help boost your self-esteem.

Journal your thoughts and feelings.

Stop negative self-talk.

Pray.

Build your strengths.

Reach out and find someone who gets it.

Focus on the positive.

Practice self-compassion.

Have gratitude.

Find humor in life where you can.

Smile. ☺

Ask for help, find the helpers.

Set boundaries and standards of how you want to be treated.
Surround yourself with goodness.
Find JOY especially on challenging days.
Tell yourself you are doing a great job!
Listen to music that feels good.

Below are just a few of Early Intervention Daily Notes from therapists that I've kept. After each home session, they would make a record of what had occurred, including any progress.

5/19/08

- Tuned people out while playing with trains
- Didn't respond to questions or his name while playing with trains; more responsive playing with playdoh and puzzles.
- Mom discussed severe aggression with therapist.
- He was leaving bruises, biting and scratching every day. Mom reported it's a severe problem. He was hurting and biting mom, dad, grandmother, and children at the library and school.
- Therapist referred OT to come look at sensory issues.

6/3/08

- Used his words and asked for what he wanted.
- Play wasn't repetitive; he used his trains purposefully and said what he was doing.
- Discussed difficulty with public places and made it a new goal.

6/10/08

- Specialist gave parents copies of IFSP and Developmental Profile. Discussed pediatrician/ specialists to assess puzzling behaviors.
- Worked with him with various toys - he got stuck on the trains. He did tantrum and perseverated (repeated actions or thoughts) through the remainder of the session.

6/25/08

- Discussed his language strengths and challenges.
- Made a plan for Mom to make social stories using photos of shopping at Walmart to help with the challenge of the items going from the cart to the cashier.
- Discussed making an eventual trip to dentist successful, introducing him to the environment.

7/2/08

- Discussed biting behavior and strategy for Mom to protect herself and interrupt the behavior. Suggested covering legs and forearms with ace bandages and put padding on thighs.
- He enjoyed puzzles, crayons, his cars and trains.
- Used a variety of toys appropriately throughout the session.

7/18/2008 -1st day of a Guided Playgroup:

I stayed outside to observe outside the room and peered through the glass. The lead teacher was wonderful.

- Dylan had a very difficult time at playgroup.
- Pushed children, hit a child, and was very aggressive.
- Mom took him out into the hall and gave him an immediate timeout but there wasn't an isolated place. He had difficulty because of space. Dylan bit her 3x. Franca came into the hallway to assist Mom. He responded to her redirection. He was over-stimulated in the play group. At first, he was clinging to Mom's leg, then biting her.

After the timeout and cooling off, he resumed to playgroup and turned around his behavior. He participated; ate snack nicely.

- Discussed Augmentative Communication with Mom
- Dylan benefitted from deep pressure massage
- Learn to create Social Stories
- Laminate pictures, create stories about feelings, transitions, places

7/23/08

- He enjoyed pretend play and related items, initiated some actions independently.
- Plan to use "First-then" board and pics (PECS) next session.

7/30/08

- Identifying emotions through pictures was implemented. Dylan was able to associate "happy and sad" with emotions.

- SCERTS program was discussed with Mom.
- A daily board was also discussed.

8/1/08

- Had to discontinue playgroup, too aggressive.
- Will try another playgroup another time.

8/14/08

- Worked on visual schedule and emotions rings.
- Discussed biting behavior.
- Provided guidance re: Mom tracking biting behavior with ABC Chart

8/28/08

- Sat at his table and picked toys to play with from photo pix.
- Used "First-Then" board, He seems to be starting to understand it.

11/25/08

- Enjoyed big noodle bin. Imitated phrases/sentences appropriately in play to narrate and request. He used some sentences spontaneously and appropriately. He gets really involved in the sensory play and sometimes overexcited. One incident of throwing; he tried to bite and struggled and eventually was guided to complete task.

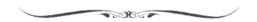

Journal your thoughts and feelings about the day you received your child's autism diagnosis. How are you processing it all?

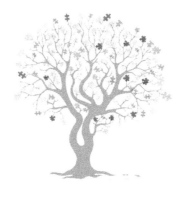

3

Your Journey to New Beginnings

"One of the most priceless gifts you can
give your children is your ability to truly see
who they are in their essence and allow
space for this to thrive."

—Dr. Shefali Tsabary

As mentioned in the last chapter, after learning
Dylan had autism my husband and I went through
a challenging period of adjustment. It was not
unlike the Five Stages of Grief: denial, anger, bargain-
ing, depression and, finally, acceptance. It was through
a combination of proper education, perseverance, hard
work and, of course, a powerful love for our son that we
were able to move forward, continue to learn and grow as
a family, and help Dylan thrive.

As a parent of a child on the spectrum, you know that life doesn't stop while you go through this process. Each day is an opportunity for them to grow, and no matter how you are feeling your first priority is to do everything you can to facilitate that. Fortunately, there are several resources, including government agencies and in-home and school-based programs, that can assist you in understanding the unique way in which your child learns and sees the world. These services can and will give you the tools to help your child develop and become more able to live an enjoyable, fulfilling life. However, you must be proactive and take advantage of these resources, even on days when you feel you are struggling to keep your head above water.

For example, if you suspect your child has developmental delays, seek a professional opinion sooner rather than later. Every day counts when it comes to the first few years of a child's development, and I strongly believe that Dylan developed the way he has because he had help early on.

As parents, we don't want to see things that may be "wrong" with our children, and we tell ourselves that it's "just a phase" and he or she will "grow out of it." You may be right, but it never hurts to get a second opinion. Start the process as soon as you can. Also, don't waste time waiting for an official diagnosis; if you suspect your child has needs that are not being met, put them in place. Think of Early Intervention as the early detection of any health issue. Time is of the essence and getting help as soon as possible can yield benefits that last a lifetime.

I cannot emphasize enough the importance of educating yourself. Learn all you can, for the more you know the better you can connect with your child and understand what they need to succeed. There are many ways you can do this. I devoured every book I could find on Autism Spectrum Disorder, and they helped tremendously. Also, join groups and ask questions. You can find local meetups and support groups, as well as many online groups and platforms such as Facebook on which to post your questions and answer those of others as you become more informed. Keep the lines of communication with your spouse or partner open to make sure you're on the same page. Be involved and learn together so you can discuss and make more informed decisions about treatment options that are right for your child.

Become an expert on your own child by meeting them where they stand. Get to know them inside and out – what their triggers are, what is easy and what is hard for them. What are their preferred activities and what activities cause disruptive behavior? What causes them stress or to become frightened? What is soothing to them? How can you calm them when they are feeling out of control? The better you know your child and how they learn, the better you will become at adjusting treatments as they develop. Remember, this is not a one-treatment-fits-all situation. It is a spectrum, so every child will have different triggers, behaviors and preferred activities that will likely change as they grow and evolve. Your role is to discover them, and to keep in mind that this is an ongoing learning process for both of you.

Accept, nurture and love your child for who they are. From the very beginning, Anthony and I loved Dylan's silly and sometimes quirky behaviors. For example, he was hypersensitive to sounds when he was learning to communicate and starting to talk. Each time he heard something different he would ask, "What's that?" over and over. One day my husband and I joked that it was like a superpower, and then we realized it was not really a joke at all. It *was* one of his superpowers, because it's what made him Dylan! From that day on we never looked at his diagnosis as a "disability," but rather an ability that gave him his unique gifts. Your child also has his or her own superpowers, so place your focus on discovering them, rather than on what they may be "lacking" in comparison to a child who is not on the spectrum. When you practice unconditional love and acceptance, your child will feel it and it will undoubtedly help their development.

Find the strength to keep moving forward. It is not easy raising a child that needs attention 24/7, but as daunting as it seems now, staying the course will be worth it for all of you in the long run. It is not possible to predict the exact outcomes, and for many parents that uncertainty is the most difficult thing. Know this: no parent knows or can control the future, whether their child is on the spectrum or not. The key is to stay positive because that will always influence outcome for the better. Don't self-sabotage by drawing conclusions about what life could be like down the road. Take one day at a time. Celebrate the little wins, and regularly look back to see how far you have come. This will keep you motivated and encouraged even during the challenging times. Mostly importantly, keep in mind that children with autism can grow up to live very fulfilling and productive lives. (This goes back to my earlier advice about educating yourself.) Many have talents that are hyper-focused, which can give them advantages others don't have. Their uniqueness helps make the world we live in that much better.

Finally, you must be diligent about setting aside time for self-care. Easier said than done, I know. It will often seem like there aren't enough hours in the day and that you don't have one more drop of energy, especially for yourself. I hear you. What you must understand though is that having a physically and emotionally strong role model is just as important for a child on the spectrum as it is for any other. They will watch and learn from your behavior, just in their own way. A tip we were given is to mirror the behavior you want your child to have and provide learning opportunities in those moments. If you can learn to cultivate calm and patience even in the most challenging situations, you will be giving one of the most powerful gifts you can to your child. That said, you must be taking care of yourself so you are not trying to give from an empty cup.

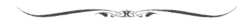

Which of your child's strengths and qualities do you love most?

_____

_____

_____

_____

_____

_____

_____

_____

_____

_____

_____

How do you celebrate your family wins?

_____

_____

_____

_____

_____

_____

_____

_____

_____

_____

_____

_____

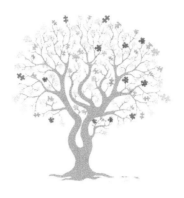

4

ABA and DIR Floortime

"Stop thinking about what could go wrong,
and start being excited about what could go right."

— Unknown

Let the Fun and Learning Begin

After a lengthy process we were finally assigned an ABA (Applied Behavioral Analysis) therapist. His name was Brendan, and I'll never forget how I felt – a combination of excitement and nervousness – before he showed up for that first appointment. As always, Karen had been a godsend, taking the time to speak to us about the therapy and minimize our uncertainty. She explained that ABA was going to be difficult – sometimes even upsetting – to observe, but that the long-term rewards would be significant.

Brendan's agency had also been extremely informative, which was one of the main reasons we chose them. During the interview they not only explained their services in detail, they were willing to answer my questions in terms I could understand. They also encouraged me to be present so I could learn about and implement what Dylan was taught after the therapists were gone. I was so desperate to understand Dylan, the way he was thinking and how I could learn to help him.

We set aside the first five minutes of each day so the therapists could answer any questions I had. I also wrote down the exercises and goals for the day and would continually ask how he was progressing. There were many days when, while Dylan napped, I sat with my notebook, writing down the phrases and terminology that Brendan had used. I would then share this information with Anthony when he was working from home or after dinner while Dylan played. It was easier to learn together, though, so whenever his work schedule allowed Anthony would stay home and observe the sessions with me.

As with everything else to that point, Anthony and I faced a learning curve when it came to ABA. Though we scheduled his sessions for times when he wouldn't be tired or hungry so he could have an optimal experience, there were still days when he screamed and cried because he did not want to participate. Of course, as a parent your first reaction is to comfort your child, but we learned quickly that this would not help him in the long run. We had to stay back and let him and Brendan work it out, and somehow they always did. Brendan was calm, kind and gentle but firm, and we knew Dylan was always in good hands.

ABA Therapy

In the beginning, the sessions were so hard to observe. Though Brendan started with very basic exercises, there were many times when Dylan refused to follow a specific direction. I would stand back and silently cry, reminding myself that Karen had warned us about this and praying he'd quickly catch on.

One of our initial goals was to get Dylan to make eye contact. Brendan would call his name, and if Dylan made eye contact he would be allowed to play with a "highly preferred" toy or some other reward. It took a few sessions to understand and trust myself with using the new language Brendan suggested because it was so foreign. Anthony learned

Antecedent - Behavior – Consequence (ABC CHART)

Name: _____ Date:_____

Target Behavior 1: _____

Target Behavior 2:_____

Target Behavior 3:_____

Target Behavior 4:_____

Intensity Score: 1= mild, 2= Moderate, 3=Extreme

Date	Time	ANTECEDENT	Location	BEHAVIOR	Int. Score	CONSEQUENCE	Initials

(ABC Antecedent, Behavior and Consequence Chart)

the language and techniques very quickly and we would practice with each other.

One particular Monday morning, Brendan showed up for our eight o'clock session excited to introduce me to The ABC (Antecedent, Behavior and Consequence) Chart. It would turn out to be a game-changer; in fact, I still use it to this day.

I strongly believe that there's a reason for every (unwanted) behavior; the key is to find it. When Dylan exhibited a specific behavior I would immediately think back to what had happened just *before* that behavior; that way I could put the pieces together to provide a learning experience and, if necessary, a consequence. My husband and I refer to it as "peeling back the onion."

Children with ASD often exhibit aggressive behaviors such as hitting, kicking, biting, and throwing objects, which can disrupt the family dynamic and cause a lot of stress. As mentioned earlier, I was often on the receiving end of Dylan's tantrums and can attest to how painful this is, both physically and emotionally.

That said, no two individuals with autism are the same and their unique personalities, coupled with the various ways in which the disorder manifests, can make things tricky. You can find tons of great information, tips and strategies for teaching self-regulation; speech and language improvement; and managing aggressive behavior and emotions; however, what works for one child may not work for another. At times, it can feel like a never-ending cycle of trial and error, leading to feelings of overwhelm and desperation. To make matters worse, others who witness the result of a less successful strategy (i.e. when your child exhibits aggressive behavior in public) are often quick to judge and offer their advice and opinions on how you should be parenting. Unless you're living it each and every day, it is not easy to understand that traditional forms of discipline may not be effective. In fact, there were many times when even I couldn't understand why Dylan wasn't making the connection between his behavior and the consequences Anthony and I were trying to implement.

Take heart! Disciplining a child with ASD is possible with the right strategies. First, though you must determine whether your child is acting out because of autism or good old age-appropriate (mis)behavior. Over the years I have struggled with this question many times; I have even reached out to friends with kiddos of the same age and asked for their opinion. That all changed when Brendan introduced us to the ABC Chart.

Below, I'll get into the specifics of ABA therapy and why it was the best option for Dylan.

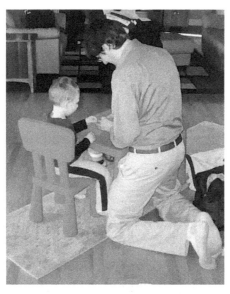

(Brendan and Dylan, ABA therapy)

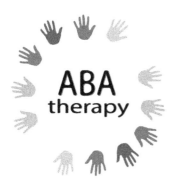

What is ABA -Applied Behavioral Analysis?

The Antecedent, Behavior, Consequence (ABC) Model is based on the science of learning and behavior. Behavior analysis helps us to understand how behavior works, how behavior is affected by the environment, and how to apply that understanding to real situations. It can be used to help individuals examine behaviors they want to change, the triggers of those behaviors, and the impact of those behaviors on negative or maladaptive patterns. The goal is to increase behaviors that are helpful and decrease behaviors that are harmful or affect learning. ABA therapy programs can also help increase language and communication skills, decrease problem behaviors, improve attention, focus, social skills, memory, and academics.

The ABC data form is an assessment tool used to gather information that should evolve into a positive behavior support plan. In essence, it provides a higher understanding of the behavior and can tell you whether it is the result of something outside your child's control (ex. sensory sensitivities) or if he or she is simply being a child and acting out.

Here are some helpful terms to understand with regard to ABA therapy:

Antecedent: Also known as a "trigger," this is the event, action, or circumstances that occurred *before* the child engaged in the target behavior. An antecedent may come from another person, such as a verbal command or request, or from the environment, such as a light, sound, toy or other object. It may also be internal, such as a thought or feeling. Some also refer to this as the "setting event."

Behavior: This refers to the particular behavior being examined. It can be verbal or an action, and it can be a pivotal, positive or problem behavior. Though it is usually in response to the antecedent, it can also indicate a *lack* of response.

Consequence: This is the *action* or *response* that follows the behavior to either encourage/discourage it moving forward. It can include positive reinforcement of the desired behavior, or no reaction for incorrect/inappropriate responses. The consequence is one of the most important elements, as it is capable of either prolonging or ending the behavior. For example, many parents tend to quiet their child by offering toys or sweets, but this only enforces the behavior they are trying to end. That said, *positive reinforcement* is one of the main strategies used in ABA. When a behavior is followed by something that is valued (a reward), a person is more likely to repeat that behavior, and over time, builds positive habits.

The idea with ABA is to trace an identical poor behavior multiple times to see if there are any consistencies in the antecedent; this will enable you to formulate a strategy to alter that event and/or consequence to make sure that behavior is extinguished. It is therefore critical that you record undesirable behavior on the ABC form every time it occurs.

ABA involves many techniques for understanding and changing behavior. It is a flexible treatment that can be adapted to meet the needs of each unique person and can be provided in different locations – home, school and out in the community. ABA teaches skills that are useful in everyday life and can involve one-on-one teaching or group instruction.

First, the therapist identifies a goal behavior. Each time the person uses the behavior or skill successfully, they get a reward. The reward is meaningful to the individual – examples include praise, a toy or book, watching a video, access to playground or other location, and more. Positive rewards encourage the person to continue using the skill. Over time this leads to meaningful behavior change.

> Children on the spectrum often do something "right" by accident or without knowing. **Positive Reinforcement** is a process that helps ensure that a behavior will occur again.

The following is from AutismSpeaks.org. I highly recommend utilizing this site as it contains a wealth of valuable information.

What Does an ABA Program Involve?

ABA is one of the most widely accepted therapies for children with autism spectrum disorder. It is most effective if therapy begins when children are younger than age five, although older children and even adults with ASD can benefit as well.

ABA focuses on improving specific behaviors, such as social skills, communication, reading, and academics as well as adaptive learning skills such as fine motor dexterity, hygiene, grooming, domestic capabilities, punctuality, and job competence.

ABA involves as much as forty hours a week of one-on-one therapy. Certified therapists deliver or oversee the regimen, organized around the child's individual needs. Individuals develop social skills, for instance, and learning to write a name or use the bathroom.

Good ABA programs for autism are not "one size fits all." ABA should not be viewed as a canned set of drills; rather, each program is written to meet the needs of the individual learner.

The goal of any ABA program is to help each person work on skills that will help them become more independent and successful in the short term, as well as in the future.

Planning and Ongoing Assessment

A qualified and trained behavior analyst (BCBA) designs and directly oversees the program. They customize the ABA program to each learner's skills, needs, interests, preferences and family situation.

The BCBA will start by doing a detailed assessment of each person's skills and preferences, which they will use this to write specific treatment goals. Family goals and preferences may be included too.

Treatment goals are written based on the age and ability level of the person with ASD. Goals can include many different skill areas, such as:

- Communication and language
- Social skills
- Self-care (such as showering and toileting)
- Play and leisure
- Motor skills
- Learning and academic skills

The instruction plan breaks down each of these skills into small, concrete steps. The therapist teaches each step one by one, from simple (e.g. imitating single sounds) to more complex (e.g. carrying on a conversation).

The BCBA and therapists measure progress by collecting data in each therapy session. Data helps them to monitor the person's progress toward goals on an ongoing basis.

The behavior analyst regularly meets with family members and program staff to review information about progress. They can then plan ahead and adjust teaching plans and goals as needed.

ABA Techniques and Philosophy

The instructor uses a variety of ABA procedures. Some are directed by the instructor and others are directed by the person with autism. Parents, family members and caregivers also receive training so they can support learning and skill practice throughout the day.

The person with autism will have many opportunities to learn and practice skills each day in both planned and naturally occurring situations. For instance, someone learning to greet others by saying hello may get the chance to practice this skill in the classroom with their teacher (planned) and on the playground at recess (naturally occurring).

The individual receives an abundance of positive rein-forcement for demonstrating useful skills and socially appropriate behaviors. The emphasis is on positive social interactions and enjoyable learning. The individual receives no reinforcement for behaviors that pose harm or prevent learning.

As mentioned above, ABA is effective for people of all ages. It can be used from early childhood through adulthood.

Who provides ABA services?

A board-certified behavior analyst (BCBA) provides ABA therapy services. To become a BCBA, they must:

- Earn a master's degree or PhD in psychology or behav-ior analysis
- Pass a national certification exam
- Seek a state license to practice (in some states)

ABA therapy programs also involve therapists, or registered behavior technicians (RBTs). These therapists are trained and supervised by the BCBA. They work directly with chil-dren and adults with autism to practice skills and work toward the individual goals written by the BCBA. You may hear them referred to by a few different names: behavioral therapists, line therapists, behavior tech, etc.

What is the evidence that ABA works?

ABA is considered an *evidence-based best practice treat-ment* by the US Surgeon General and by the American Psy-chological Association. ABA therapists only use teaching strategies that have been clinically proven to be effective.

"Evidence based" means that ABA has passed scientific tests of its usefulness, quality, and effectiveness. ABA therapy includes many different techniques. All of these techniques focus on antecedents (what happens before a behavior occurs) and on consequences (what happens after the behavior).

More than twenty studies have established that *intensive* and *long-term* therapy using ABA principles improves outcomes for many but not all children with autism. "Intensive" and "long term" refer to programs that provide twenty-five to forty hours a week of therapy for one to three years. These studies show gains in intellectual functioning, language development, daily living skills and social functioning. Studies with adults using ABA principles, though fewer in number, show similar benefits.

Is ABA covered by insurance?

Sometimes. Many types of private health insurance are required to cover ABA services. This depends on what kind of insurance you have, and what state you live in.

All Medicaid plans must cover treatments that are *medically necessary* for children under the age of twenty-one. If a doctor prescribes ABA and says it is medically necessary for your child, Medicaid must cover the cost.

Where do I find ABA services?

To get started, follow these steps:

- Speak with your pediatrician or other medical provider to discuss whether ABA is right for your child. They can write a prescription for ABA if it is necessary for your insurance.

- Check whether your insurance company covers the cost of ABA therapy, and what that coverage entails (i.e. your deductible).
- Search the resource directory for ABA providers near you, or ask your child's doctor and teachers for recommendations.
- Call the ABA provider and request an intake evaluation.

What questions should I ask?

An ABA therapist is a person who uses applied behavior analysis as a form of treatment. It is the process of studying behavior in order to put into place appropriate behavioral interventions. It's important to find an ABA provider and therapists who are a good fit for your family. The first step is for therapists to establish a good relationship with your child. If your child trusts his therapists and enjoys spending time with them, therapy will be more successful – and fun!

The following questions can be helpful in evaluating a provider. Remember to trust your instincts as well!

- How many BCBAs do you have on staff?
- Are they licensed with the BACB and through the state?
- How many behavioral therapists do you have?
- How many therapists will be working with my child?
- What sort of training do your therapists receive? How often?
- How much direct supervision do therapists receive from BCBAs weekly?
- How do you manage safety concerns?

- What does a typical ABA session look like?
- Do you offer home-based or clinic-based therapy?
- How do you determine goals for my child? Do you consider input from parents?
- How often do you re-evaluate goals?
- How is progress evaluated?
- How many hours per week can you provide?
- Do you have a wait list?
- What type of insurance do you accept?

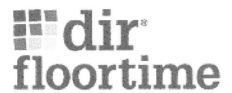 While we did not choose the DIR/Floortime Approach, I know many families who have been very successful with it as well. The following is an overview of this type of therapy.

The DIR/Floortime Approach is a developmentally-based approach that addresses the core deficits generally displayed in children with ASD (social, emotional, communication, and play skills). It focuses on helping them master the building blocks of relating, communicating and thinking, and thus relies heavily on developing a strong relationship with the child in order to motivate and foster development. It is a more child-directed approach than ABA and views parental involvement as key.

The "D" is for Developmental: understanding how your child functions developmentally is critical to planning a treatment program.

A play-based assessment is conducted to help figure out where your child is on six critical development milestones. The DIR Approach was developed by Drs. Stanley Greenspan and Serena Wieder. Some of the cornerstones of DIR include:

- Child-focused: understanding whole context
- Importance of relationship: foundation for learning
- Functional: developmentally appropriate
- Integrated
- Parent involvement
- Generalization from the beginning

The "I" is for your child's individual differences. Your child has their own way of taking in the world – sights, sounds, touch, et cetera – and responding to it.

- Does your child hear everything, even sounds that are far away?
- Do they like to be touched?
- Do they have difficulty navigating their way through space?
- Is getting them into water a challenge?
- Do they love to roughhouse and be tickled?

The "R" is for Relationship

The therapists will work hard to establish a strong relationship with your child in order to gain his or her trust. As you are an essential person in your child's life, strategies and opportunities for Floortime "coaching" will be provided so you can help further his or her development.

During Floortime, your child will lead as they engage in things that interest them. Once the therapists enter into a play relationship, they will provide many opportunities to challenge your child to communicate and relate to others socially.

Questions and Answers

- Can I participate in my child's DIR/Floortime Sessions?

  For sure! Your involvement is a critical piece in your child's development. You are encouraged to be as involved as possible.

- What will my child's DIR/Floortime sessions look like?

  This will depend on your child's particular needs. Therapists will begin by joining your child in the things they already like to do, according to his or her agenda, rather than their own. If your child has very few play skills, this may seem silly at first; however, the expectation is that by entering into your child's world they will then be able to draw them out into ours and challenge them.

- Is there a way to provide both DIR/Floortime as well as ABA to my child?

  Sure. Many children benefit from a blend of both methods – usually when various techniques based on ABA principles are incorporated into DIR. Generally, DIR/Floortime doesn't provide Discrete Trial Teaching. In the event you would like your child to receive this type of service, you could be referred to a specialty provider and work in collaboration with them.

What to Expect from Specialty Services

Once you have chosen what intervention you would like for your child, the specialist will pay visits to your home to observe your child and your interactions with him or her. The goal is to establish which functional emotional developmental milestones your child has mastered, and where intervention will be focused initially. Here are some key processes and procedures:

- The therapists will want to learn more about your child's individual differences, for example with regard to sensory sensitivities and processing capacities. They will also assess his or her relationships with others, for example, patterns within the family, including supports and challenges that affect growth.

- A developmental profile summarizing these areas and making initial recommendations for goals and strategies will be compiled.

- There will be a coordination meeting in your home with specialty services staff and early intervention staff prior to beginning. The purpose of this meeting is to discuss the developmental profile and agree on the goals to review your child's progress and assess gains made throughout the intervention. Recommendations will be made at this point as to whether to modify your child's program. They will also discuss the suitability for the number of hours in which your child will be receiving.

- Quarterly meetings will be to assess progress and modify goals and strategies needed.

- Therapists will compile a final report summarizing your child's progress and make recommendations to help your child continue to grow as he or she enters the school system.

(What is the DIR Floortime Approach, Autism Specialty Service, REACH Program, MA)

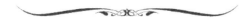

Journal how Behavioral Therapy is going for your child.

What goals have been met or are a work in progress?

_____

_____

_____

_____

_____

_____

_____

_____

_____

_____

_____

Are you happy with how things are going?

_____

_____

_____

_____

_____

_____

_____

_____

_____

_____

_____

_____

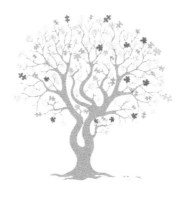

5

The 3 C's Connection, Communication and Conversation

"Just because your child isn't communicating verbally, doesn't mean they aren't communicating."

—Nicole Lusardi

As mentioned earlier, when Dylan started Early Intervention he was acting out in ways that were shocking, confusing and concerning: biting, hitting, banging his head and crying any time we transitioned from one activity to another. Indeed, this was one of the reasons we had him evaluated in the first place. As much as we wanted to believe that this was within the acceptable range of childhood behavior, we couldn't deny that a simple trip to the market had become a major challenge, with Dylan melting down as we left the house, got into and out of the car, entered the store, placed items on the counter to pay and returned to the car. It wasn't until EI started that we learned that with each and every behavior Dylan was actually communicating something.

Anthony and I did our best to meet his needs. I purchased a shopping cart cover so he was comfortable when I planned to have him sit in the shopping cart. I always brought along a couple of "highly preferred" toys, a sippy cup, snacks and a sensory oral toy to distract him, but it never went as planned. Clearly I was missing something.

After many such attempts, I started waiting until Anthony could watch Dylan while I ran out to do errands. I also spoke to the EI Coordinator about the situation, and when I told her that I wanted to bring Dylan shopping with me, that once each meltdown had passed I genuinely enjoyed our time together, she suggested I ask the OT about ways to better handle transitions. Though their advice was excellent, it took perseverance and patience to implement it. Each morning, after Early Intervention services were over, I struggled to transition him in the car. Once I was able to secure him in his car seat safely, I put on soft music and started singing to him. It worked! As we drove around Dylan grew more and more relaxed until he fell asleep, and I enjoyed seeing him calm and having quiet time. Excited, I decided to continue this "experiment" until his next appointment with the OT and I could ask for additional ideas.

It was on one of the rides that I made another discovery – coffee! Of course I knew what it was, but I had never been a coffee drinker. That day, I passed a coffeehouse with a drive-thru window and suddenly got the urge to go. In the back, Dylan was still asleep and comfortable, so I pulled up to the window and ordered myself an iced coffee. It was heavenly, and the perfect way to celebrate my victory. I had finally found a way to have quiet time *out of the house* and with Dylan!

On other days, I'd bring a book or my binder so I could catch up with my notes. Sometimes I would just stare into the sky with tired eyes. Encouraged by this success, the OT came up with a truly brilliant idea: she would accompany me and Dylan on a trip to Target to see how he did. When I explained that when we went I stayed on the perimeter of the store where there weren't as many people, she said this first time would be an experiment, a chance for her to observe the meltdowns and their triggers such as sights, sounds and lights.

After that trip she had many helpful ideas and suggestions – the top one being that I create Visual Social Stories and Visual Schedules for *all* transitions. At the time, I was only taking Dylan to Target and the grocery store, so those were the locations I focused on. One evening I went out by myself and took photos of my car, the parking lots of both stores, the signs on the buildings, a few as I entered the cashier area and down some of the aisles. I kept the photos simple so when I created the Social Stories it would be easy for him to follow along. I purchased laminating paper and printed out the photos, then punched holes in them and bound them together with a ring to create the story. I'll always remember how excited I felt as I presented the Social Stories to Dylan. We went over them many times, then started with Target, and after practicing for a few weeks, we moved on to the grocery store. It was a SUCCESS!

The ABA therapist and SLP also taught and encouraged Dylan how to use picture cards to communicate. When everyone was on the same page and his schedule was consistent, we recognized the positive changes. Dylan would point to the things he wanted – juice, cereal, or a toy, for example. We noticed that the frequency of his outbursts slowly decreased. The strict set routine helped us, and helped him to know what was coming each time, each moment, each hour. We created rituals, with the same naptimes and bedtimes, watching the same videos for the hundredth time, and reading to him every night. Life began to shine brighter.

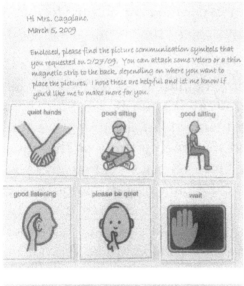
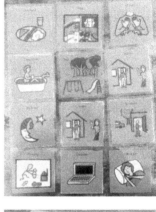
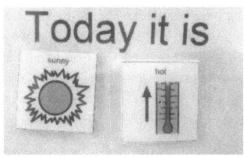
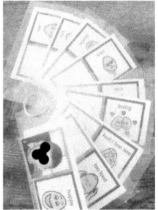

(Examples of picture icons and symbols of feelings,
places and common phrases)

As Dylan's needs changed and he grew, so did the Visual and Social Stories I made. Below are examples of additional symbol photos, provided by EI during that time. You can make them yourself by going on Pinterest, Shutter Stock and other sites, where you'll find free printable photos for Visual Picture Schedules and free clip art for Social Stories.

Visual Schedules

Visual schedules are great for children who thrive on routine and predictability and can be used at home and in school for consistency. They are often arranged to sequence activities by using photos or words. They help set expectations at the beginning of the day and can be extremely effective in decreasing unwanted behavior, as they help children who get "stuck" on and act out in response to schedule changes. Preparing them ahead of time allows children to move from one activity to the next without prompting and increases their motivation to complete less desired tasks. Dylan thrived using his visual schedule which lessened his

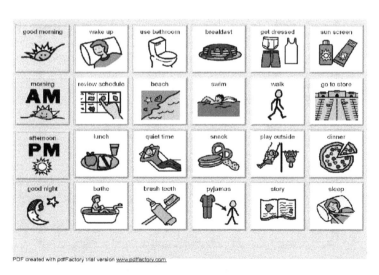

(Example of a visual schedule)

frustration significantly. Actually, this is no different from adults, as we use visual schedules to add structure to our lives by using a calendar, sticky notes, or a daily to-do list.

Sign Language

Sign language is a visual mode of communication most commonly associated with the hearing impaired; as we soon learned, however, it is extremely beneficial for children with ASD as well. Twenty years of scientific research bears this out, providing evidence of social, emotional, communicative

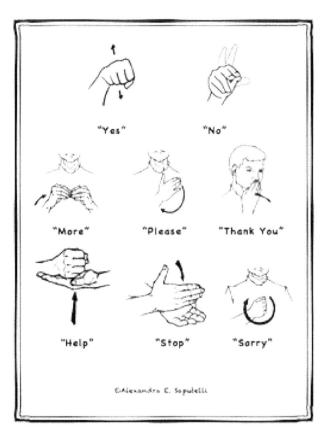

(Example of sign language)

and cognitive improvements. Sign language can reduce negative social behaviors such as anxiety, self-injury, tantrums and aggression, which often intensify when a child cannot communicate their basic wants and needs. Learning sign language allows a child to express themselves clearly, which boosts their self-esteem and emotional development. In an effort to decrease Dylan's frustration and the resulting biting and other behaviors, the SLP suggested we learn to sign. Anthony and I tried to be open to all of EI's suggestions; we needed all the hope we could get and certainly had nothing to lose by trying it. We started with the basics, such as feelings, common phrases, food, toys, and objects that were familiar to him, and found it to be very effective.

Change of Plans

One day, Anthony and I decided to take Dylan to the park. After putting the visual schedule together and priming Dylan, we excitedly headed out only to find that the park was *closed*! I remember feeling panicked because I had planned ahead and prepared him, explained the visual schedule, spoke about it for transitioning purposes, and then boom!

The next day I spoke to the therapist about it. She told me that just as I had prepared Dylan for transitions, I could prepare him for unexpected situations such as this. She then provided a couple "what if" situations. What if the park is closed again? What if the seat you want is taken when you go to a new place or restaurant? What if you can't find the show he usually watches? This was exactly the support I needed. Though I was doing everything I could to make things just right for him – and avoid those meltdowns – I was constantly anxious and nervous, always thinking everything might fall apart. I realized I could plan and schedule all I wanted, but life happens! I didn't want to be afraid to go out in public. I wanted to feel secure in my words and actions when an incident occurred.

The therapist explained that it was going to take time for Dylan to adjust to this new teaching, and that I needed to be structured but more flexible. I found that balance to be a struggle, and so to lighten the mood Anthony and I started to call each trip out of the house a "field trip." We soon realized that the more we practiced going on "field trips" the better Dylan did. We would fill the backpack with highly preferred items such as juice, snacks, toys, sensory tools, and so on, then I would talk about the trip and prime him with the Visual Schedule on the way to where we were going. After that I had to just let it go and hope for the best outcome.

When we arrived back home, we would try to take a few minutes to recap or wrap up the "field trip" with Dylan and offer positive praise. For example, I would say something like, "We went to the grocery store. I know it's not your favorite place because of the noise and lights. You did a great job looking at me when I asked you questions. Great job listening."

On the occasions when either I or Anthony took him out alone, we would fill each other in then reiterate it in order to encourage Dylan. For example, "Dad told me you did a great job standing in line and listening when he was ready to leave the store," or "Mom told me you walked to the car nicely when you left the park." The positive praise and feedback helped build his confidence and we would use the positive moments to lay the foundation for future successful trips.

Dylan never knew how to instinctively act in a public place, know how to greet someone, or play with a new friend. He had to be taught every skill, idea and concept he knows, and he continues to learn on a daily basis.

Every day I tried different ways to connect and communicate with Dylan. It was something I had to learn and practice. If I asked him two questions he would always respond only to the second question; he didn't even hear the first. We found that so interesting. Individuals with ASD often appear to understand more than they actually do. At times, they can repeat back what they hear without understanding. Verbalizing words does not equal comprehension.

We found it was imperative to get Dylan's attention *before* trying to speak to him, especially if he was in a different room or playing with something highly preferred. We did this by saying his name to him and getting his eye contact. One statement we found particularly helpful at the time was, "If the child understands individual words this does not mean that he/she understands those words in a sentence." Keep this in mind and if your child doesn't understand what you're saying, try asking questions in different ways and keep sentences short and precise.

Learning to communicate clearly and concisely was one of the important, and most challenging, things that Anthony and I had to do. Again, the visuals were incredibly helpful. Our goal was to teach life skills – how to communicate with words and how to dress, brush his teeth, potty train, et cetera; therefore, when Dylan's language and speech skills began to emerge the SLP suggested we label everything in our kitchen, bathroom, playroom and living room. She also explained the benefits of talking through activities, to tell him about every step of my daily household routine while, as mentioned, trying to keep our words brief and precise.

It was an exhausting time for sure, but incredibly effective in the long run. "Dylan, (the first part was having his attention and looking at me), Mommy is pouring the juice into the cup. Mommy is opening the refrigerator and putting away the juice. Dylan, here is your sippy cup to drink your juice." I would go through the day and talk out loud about everything I did. Looking back, it was time-consuming and I was tired, but the payoff was well worth it. Once we had his attention and we were doing the work the therapists had taught us to do when they were gone, we started to see real growth. He would try to use his words, imitate language to request, declare or comment.

Dylan also started scripting words, phrases and movies, also known as "delayed echolalia." This is when a child has some language but is not conversational. He would repeat almost everything I said to him back to me. We were happy he was talking, but concerned it would interfere with his functional communication. It was a slow process, but with speech and ABA therapy we were able to get the echolalia under instructional control when he fully started talking. Eventually it stopped altogether.

> **Echolalia** is the repetition of phrases, words or parts of words. Almost all toddlers go through a stage in which they "parrot" words and phrases that they overhear, however, echolalia may be a sign of autism, another neurological condition, a visual impairment or a developmental disability.

Over the years, we have learned that when we present an idea to Dylan in a positive, upbeat fashion and as long as he knows what's coming or where he's going ahead of time, we've likely set him up for a successful transition. Of course, there have been some bumps in the road. I remember one particular "field trip" to Target when, as I began setting up the shopping cart cover for his comfort, Dylan began biting my arm and head bunting me. As often as this happened I was never ready for it and it caught me off guard. My only goal was to keep him safe and sometimes that meant holding him (the way EI showed me to) so he didn't continue to hurt me or himself. As I calmly but firmly told him to stop the behavior I did not know I was being watched by a woman in a car parked across from me. She saw my struggle but didn't ask if she could help. Instead, she called the police.

When I saw the officer walking toward us I was horrified. He was very nice, and when I explained the situation he asked what he could do. He opened my minivan, then helped me put Dylan back in his car seat. Before he left, he offered a great tip incase this ever happened again: *keep a copy of his official diagnosis in the glove compartment.*

The woman left before he or I could approach her. Though part of me was angry, I was also grateful that she cared enough to make the call. I cried all the way home, filled with a mix of self-consciousness and worry that this could happen again in the future. What I wish I knew then is that there is no guilt to be had or blame to be placed. There is nothing I could have done differently to prevent Dylan's diagnosis.

(Public Autism Awareness Card, AutismSociety.org)

When your child melts down, or engages in stereotypical autistic behaviors in public, there is a good chance you will receive stares. I was not prepared for this, but I did find a way to work through the problem when it came up. I ordered "Autism Awareness Cards" from the Autism Society and handed them out to family, friends and strangers alike. I wanted to educate as many folks as I could. Often there were questions, but mostly awkward silences. I quickly learned there are people who "know everything about parenting" and feel the need to offer "advice" and say hurtful things without thinking. Everyone, no matter where you turn, will have ideas or suggestions about what you should be doing. I believe people genuinely don't know what to say and are trying to be helpful; their delivery is just off. My advice: *Stay in your own lane, let it go, be confident in your choices, you're doing a great job!*

Below are some tips provided to us by our SLP when Dylan was diagnosed. They are for promoting language development in nonverbal individuals with autism and we found them very helpful.

Encourage play and social interaction. Most children learn through play, including those with ASD. Learning the basics of language through interacting and play is meaningful. Try a variety of games (you can search many on Pinterest) that your child will enjoy. Include playful activities that promote social interaction, for example, singing and reciting nursery rhymes.

Get their attention. Sit in front of your child and close to eye level. You can encourage eye contact by holding a favorite toy or object near your eye. Hold it there and wait for them to look at you before giving it to them. This is a great way to get your child's full attention and will make it easier for them to see, hear and connect with you.

Imitate your child. Before children learn to copy words and talk, they learn to copy gestures and movements. Mimicking your child's sounds and play behaviors will encourage more vocalizing and interaction. It also encourages him or her to copy you and take turns. Be sure to always use positive behavior and an upbeat tone of voice.

Focus on nonverbal communication. Communication doesn't always refer to speaking, but it's still important to speak with a nonverbal child. Keep it short (using one word) and talk about what your child is doing. Children with ASD are often unable to use gestures, such as pointing to an object, to give meaning to their speech. They will also often avoid eye contact, which can make them appear uninterested or inattentive. Pay attention to nonverbal signs, behaviors and facial expressions. Find out what works best for your child and use it regularly.

Gestures and eye contact can build a foundation for language. As mentioned above, exaggerate and model gestures that are easy to imitate by using both your body and your voice. Also, if they say a sound or word, repeat it back to them. Copying them will help them learn how to copy you and take turns.

Leave "space" for your child to talk and pick the right moments. When a child doesn't immediately respond, it's natural as a parent to start talking and fill in the language. It's important to give your child opportunities to communicate, even if he or she isn't talking. When you ask a question or see that your child wants something, pause for several seconds and continue looking at them. Do you see any body movement or hear any sounds? If so, respond quickly. Your response helps your child feel the power of communication.

Finding the right time to talk with your child is important because of their particular schedules. If you find he/she is occupied with something else and you interrupt that time, you may not get the response you hoped for. Be patient and wait for a calm moment to talk.

Simplify your language and keep it to the point. Whenever possible, be short, simple, and direct. This helps your child to follow what you're saying. Stay away from allusions, metaphors, or any abstract statements. Children with autism often will not be able to read your body language or read your emotions. Try to keep the pace of the conversation at a level the child can maintain. Children with autism need more time to work out what they hear.

Try writing if speaking isn't working. ASD children tend to think visually. Drawing a picture or writing down the words on paper can be very helpful.

Follow your child's interests and talk about them. Rather than interrupting your child's focus, follow along with words. Talk about what engages your child, their highly preferred topics and related ideas. Trying to have a conversation of your choice may not go in the direction you hoped for. You may get ignored, or your child may have a meltdown or shut down altogether.

Consider assistive devices and visual supports. Assistive technologies and visual supports can do more than take the place of speech. They can foster development. Use devices and apps with pictures that your child touches to produce words. Visual supports can include pictures, social stories, or groups of pictures that your child can use to indicate requests and thoughts.

Keep good communication with your child's therapists. By working with your child's EI team, you can help provide the support your child needs to find his or her unique "voice." You are their best advocate for success.

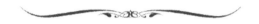

How does your child communicate with you?

_____

_____

_____

_____

_____

_____

_____

_____

_____

_____

_____

What goals are you working on?

_____

_____

_____

_____

_____

_____

_____

_____

_____

_____

_____

_____

_____

Tips for Connection, Communication and Conversation

- Be patient, flexible and kind.
- Be persistent yet resilient.
- Be in the moment.
- Stay positive.
- Protect yourself if they display (unwanted) behaviors towards you.
- Ignore attention-seeking behavior.
- Be affectionate and show interest in ways they prefer/allow.
- Use positive reinforcement and praise.
- Don't take responses personally if they're blunt and hurtful.
- Make sure your child is relaxed and you feel they're ready to talk with you. Timing is everything. Turn off distractions (tv, music, toys, etc.) so they focus on you. Give them your full attention.
- Use simple language, gestures, or other non-verbal ways to communicate. Ask one question at a time and wait patiently for their response so they feel heard. Follow up with questions based on their answers to keep the conversation going. Find ways to reach your child.
- Get creative and be inspired by what is important to him/her. Show a picture or social story of something fun you did together and ask your child about it. Point out something you've noticed and ask questions about

the specific object. Know when to stop the conversation when you feel your child is done talking. Try to choose a topic that will spark their interest.

- If you've asked a question without receiving a response, try again. If you have to ask a third time, consider rephrasing the question using different words. Consider using pictures and have them point.

- Have FUN together and make memories! ☺

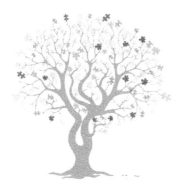

6

The Verbal Behavior Approach with Dr. Mary Barbera

"My advice is: You always have to
keep persevering."

—Dr. Temple Grandin

I'd like to share an AMAZING resource with you. Her name is Dr. Mary Barbera and her passion is helping parents of individuals with autism and the professionals who work with them. She is also an autism mom herself. Dr. Barbera has been a Board Certified Behavior Analyst (BCBA) since 2003, and in 2010 she developed her own procedures to help children who were not talking, talking minimally, or with "pop out" words. Her book, *The Verbal Behavior Approach* (which is a form of Applied Behavioral Analysis (ABA)), is an easy to read, step-by-step

guide for parents. It offers a wealth of invaluable information without being overwhelming, as do her courses and
weekly podcasts. Everything can be found on her website,
www.marybarbera.com.

Each week, Dr. Barbera offers innovative ideas on her podcasts and YouTube channel, and I always learn something
useful. For example, in her July 24, 2019 episode, "Increas-
ing Language in Children with Autism through a Shoebox,"
she discusses the "shoebox procedure," which she created
while working with one-, two-, and three-year-olds, to help
parents elicit more language from their child. She also does
a great job of explaining mand and request of your child and
how it applies to ABA. (Early mand/request training is a form
of behavioral training that uses prompting and reinforcement of requests to get preferred items or activities. This is
the first step in teaching language, as it is based upon student motivation and results in a student being reinforced,
specifically with regard to what he/she has requested.). She
also explains the language, including terms like "echoic
control," in a way that parents can understand.

Here are five quick strategies she explains in the video:

1. Look at the entire situation and do a full assessment.

She believes in meeting the child where they are, not just
with respect to speech, but the whole person. For example,
how old is the child? Can comprehend simple directions?
Touch the correct body parts when asked? Other factors to
consider are whether they have allergies and if they have a
diagnosis or are waiting for one. She also discusses feeding
issues, for as she states, "I can almost guarantee there will
be problems with eating and drinking as well," and speech

problems. Do they have problems with the mushy foods, finger foods? Do they refuse utensils? Are they addicted to a pacifier or a bottle or a spill-proof sippy cup? Are there major problem behaviors during feedings?

2. Carefully assess the child's talking abilities.

Are they really nonverbal? If they do speak, do they have word approximation? If not, are they making sounds? Even if the child just has a couple of words (which she refers to as "pop out" words) with poor articulation, Dr. Barbera believes you can, using certain techniques, get these words under "echoic control," which means "I say ball, you say ball."

3. Assess where they are and, if necessary, stop talking in sentences and using carrier phrases.

Slow down your speech and focus on one- or two-syllable words. Choose words important to the child, for example, mama, cookie, drink, juice, milk. Slow down and use more energy in your talking, for example, "Johnny, let's go up the steps to get a bath." If your child doesn't understand this, try saying "Up! Up! Up!" in a playful and animated tone. The key is to emphasize one word as you're climbing the steps. That may make a difference and you may start to hear more words.

4. Use easy materials like a potato head or a shoebox.

The Shoebox Method: cut a slit into the top of the shoebox and choose pictures important to the child (i.e. of Mommy, Daddy, car, ball, sun, dog, etc.). Collect the pictures or take them yourself. You can also buy flashcards with pictures on them. Then, say the word slowly and in an animated tone. Continue to make it fun and have the child *put each picture in the box.*

Dr. Barbera discusses the blurry lines between high-functioning and low-functioning autism. "Focus on a child reaching their full potential, instead of the type of autism they have." In other words, focus on using their strengths to bring up their weaknesses and improve those deficits to help each child be as safe, independent and happy as possible. When children are really young, newly diagnosed or waiting to be diagnosed, it's impossible to know how they will do long term.

"You need to treat early autism like the worst case of autism you've ever seen in order to give your child the best outcome possible."

–Dr. Mary Barbera

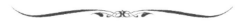

Journal your thoughts on how implementing Behavior Therapy in your child's life has helped him or her.

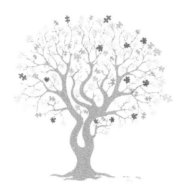

7

Tantrums and Meltdowns

"All kids need is a little help,
a little hope, and someone who believes in them."
—Magic Johnson

As you've read throughout this book, the struggle of tantrums and meltdowns in our house was REAL. These moments were extremely intense and it took a lot of work for me and Anthony to learn to manage them. Knowing there is no such thing as a one-size-fits-all approach, we tried a variety of suggestions from behavioral therapists. The key, we realized, was to stay strong together, though to be honest there were times when we weren't on the same page, which only added to the issue at hand.

Though we had been dealing with tantrums and meltdowns for some time, we didn't realize there are actually differences between the two. Even after Brendan and the EI team explained this it was hard for us to differentiate because the behaviors look so similar. It was only after we gained greater awareness of the underlying triggers that we were able to respond in ways that helped Dylan regain control.

Tantrum is an outburst that happens when kids are trying to get something they want or need. Tantrums have a purpose.

Meltdown is a reaction to feeling overwhelmed and a result of sensory overload.

As noted above, the main difference between tantrums and meltdowns is that tantrums usually have a purpose and meltdowns are usually a reaction to something. A temper tantrum usually occurs when a child is denied what they want to do or what they want to have – in other words, the type of behavior one normally categories as the "terrible twos." At this age, children are beginning to assert independence and develop problem-solving skills. They are engaging in this behavior because they believe on some level that it will get them what they want.

That is not the case with meltdowns, though. When a child has a meltdown, he or she is reacting to some sort of stimuli that is out of their control. A meltdown can end in a couple different ways. The first is fatigue, when the child finally wears themselves out. Dylan's meltdowns were intense; then his body would go limp and he would often fall sleep. The other way is a change in the amount of sensory input (noises or other stimuli in the environment) that helps the child feel less overwhelmed.

Once we were able to recognize and observe the differences between Dylan's meltdowns and tantrums, we were better able to help him through them. Here are two strategies to keep in mind:

- *When your child is having a tantrum, acknowledge what he or she wants without giving in.* Communicate clearly that you understand what your child is looking for. "I see that you want my attention. When your brother is done talking, it will be your turn." The goal is to teach your child that there are appropriate options with regard to their behavior.

- *When your child is having a meltdown, de-escalate in a safe, quiet place.* Provide a calm, supportive, reassuring presence without talking too much. The goal is to reduce how much information (i.e. noise, sight, and sound) is coming in.

You'll need different game plans depending on what kind of environment you're in, for example, the library, store, park, doctor's office, picnic at a friend's house, a family outing, and so on. These moments will still be stressful, but you can manage as a family when you have a plan.

Also, learn to let the opinions of others roll off your back. We've all seen kiddos crying in the grocery store or park. From a distance, we assume it's a tantrum, and perhaps it is, but there are many times when it's a full-fledged meltdown. When it is our child, we pray that others won't judge us, and indeed, there have been people who have offered to help right in the middle of a store. (One woman kindly offered to distract Dylan by singing!) That said, most do judge, and one of the most empowering moments in this whole journey was when I decided to just ignore the stares and comments. I just needed to find my voice instead of holding back my feelings and wanting to cry and, believe it or not, it worked!

The good news when it comes to tantrums is that kids usually have some control over them. For example, they often change their behavior based on how people around them are reacting. As mentioned earlier, this is not the case with meltdowns. Here are a few suggestions we've had success with meltdowns over the years.

Remember the ABC Chart I mentioned in Chapter 4? Well, this is exactly when you'd utilize it. What are your child's triggers? Is it pain or fear? Unexpected changes? Sensory overload or something emotional? Every child is different and the triggers are not always obvious, so you may need to keep track for a while in order to recognize the patterns. Do meltdowns occur at certain times of the day, such as before or after school? When they are hungry, tired or too excited? During transitions or when they're in a new environment? Do smells, noises or too many people set them off?

Once you can recognize that your child's behavior is escalating, you can notice the signs and de-escalate the situation prior to a full-blown meltdown. For us, redirecting Dylan's thoughts worked like a charm. Try talking about something different and starting a new activity – that was our go-to! Easier said than done, but with practice and patience you can do it. Your first instinct will be to try to stop the escalation right away, but talking loud and fast could often make things worse in the moment. Keep your sentences short and precise and allow extra time for your child to process what you are saying.

Too many times to count, the meltdown came on like a freight train and Dylan would start screaming, kicking and banging his head. Our first thought always was his safety. Through trial and error, we figured out that he benefitted from firm deep hugs and gently squeezing his arms. That said, other children need distance when they're going through this. Once again, knowing your child is key.

What are your child's warning signs?

- Refusing to follow directions or cooperate
- Trying to shut out noises, sights
- Running away or hiding
- Fidgeting or pacing
- Complaining of physical issues like dizziness or a pounding heart
- Trouble thinking clearly, making decisions, or responding to questions
- Repeating thoughts or questions over and over

When Dylan was diagnosed, the doctor gave us an analogy to keep in mind when he was melting down. Imagine your child sitting in a chair, his hands under his bottom, while someone flashes a light in his face, someone whispers in his ear, and a loud fire truck zooms by with sirens blaring. Lots of over-stimulation going on at once, right? That, she said, is how Dylan may feel. This was another a-ha moment for me. I had always been desperate to know how he was feeling inside, and this description, as disturbing as it was, provided clarity and helped me to find more grace and patience with him and myself. I was able to reassure him in a calming, soothing voice. My voice calmed me as well. Keep your voice and body language calm and use your intuition to figure out what they need from you. Be present and in the moment.

In time, you'll also develop a strategy for after the meltdown is over. Dylan was often quiet, embarrassed and exhausted afterward. I was exhausted too. At times, I'd try to gather my thoughts and document everything on the ABC chart, including what I said or did that was effective and what wasn't. Find what works for you, and give your child some space and time to collect themselves.

At some point, Anthony and I would talk things through with Dylan, which brought us closure and some comfort after the intense time. It's important to give your child a heads up that you'll be having a talk, and let them know they aren't in trouble. Keep it short and simple. Dylan often became defensive and embarrassed. It was important to us to communicate how we felt and listen to how he felt as well. We always made sure to answer his questions so he was clear about what had happened and why. As upsetting as these times were, Dylan always grew from them and we grew as a family. At the end of the day, we're all just doing the best we can. Continue to give lots of hugs, kisses (if your child allows you to) and continue giving yourselves grace.

Meltdown Tips

- Be understanding and patient. Use short, concrete sentences and give your child space and time to process what you're saying.
- Consider the environment and identify and remove sensory triggers

- Try distracting your child
- Make your child feel safe
- Remove any dangerous objects
- Invest in a good weighted blanket
- Always carry a pair of noise-cancelling headphones
- Keep an emergency meltdown backpack available
- Stay calm

What if you didn't know how to change your level of emotions? This is the case with many people with autism when they are feeling angry, scared, anxious or getting upset. Find ways to create balance in your child's day with a combination of low stress and high pleasure activities. We had an incredible OT who provided us with many ideas to help Dylan feel "grounded." Here are some options:

- Wearing a weighted vest
- Putting deep pressure on shoulders
- Using weighted blanket
- Pushing a cart or wagon
- Playing with resistive putty
- Erasing a chalk board or easel
- Carrying a weighted backpack
- Exercising
- Doing a "wheelbarrow" walk"
- Carrying toys ... to name a few!

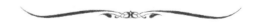

Journal the strategies that work for your child or, if you'd like, write new goals for meltdowns.

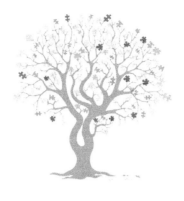

8

Discipline and Positive Parenting

"Your words as a parent have great power.
Use them wisely and
make sure they come from the heart."
—Carolina King

Having a good understanding of your child's diagnosis will be extremely helpful with regard to discipline. The autism spectrum is vast and the symptoms can vary greatly, so it's imperative that you know your child inside and out in order to set realistic expectations of their child's needs and abilities. The same is true for disciplining a child on the spectrum. There will be days and moments when we feel we are reaching our limit and need to change things fast, but the reality is that changing behavior is a process. Choosing one behavior to work on at a time will be helpful and less overwhelming. Take a few minutes to create a list of the challenges you and your child are struggling with; then pick the behavior from the list that causes the most difficulty or disruptions to your daily routine or puts you, your child, or others at risk.

A wise person once said:

> '*My child isn't* **GIVING** *me a hard time.*
> *My child is* **HAVING** *a hard time.*'

The first step is to identify the *why* behind the behavior (this is also known as getting to the root of the behavior or, as Anthony and I say, "peeling back the onion"). Whatever you call it, knowing the why is an integral part of correcting behavioral issues. For example, Dylan used to hit us to get our attention or when he wanted something. We started tracking his hitting on the ABC Chart to understand the antecedent, which helped us meet his needs more efficiently. We also taught him to use Visual Stories/Schedules, which along with the sign language helped him communicate those needs. It took several months, but the hitting behavior was eventually extinguished. This became our protocol with every unwanted behavior. It requires patience and time to practice (depending upon where they are on the spectrum your child may struggle to understand the consequences of his/her actions), but it will make a huge change in your life.

Do you have a plan in place for your child's unwanted behaviors? Here are a few suggestions, many of which you'll find are similar to those for dealing with meltdowns.

- Learn your child's triggers.
- Be consistent when dealing with behaviors.
- Plan ahead, keeping any transitions in mind; for example, what they may need when you leave the house (a highly preferred toy, a favorite drink, iPad, noise-cancelling headphones, pleasing music, etc.).
- When the world becomes overstimulating, create a safe space in public or a safety zone at home. It may take a while, but once you know what keeps your child calm and safe you will feel more equipped when a problem arises.

Positive reinforcement, or the act of rewarding a child with an incentive when he/she engages in a desired behavior, is an effective technique parents, teachers and caregivers can utilize to improve behavioral issues. For example, when you reward your child and praise them for behaving in a certain way, they are likely to do so more often. As such positive reinforcement can open the doors to functional skills and academic learning. Be diligent about pointing out when your child behaves appropriately or does something you notice when they think you aren't watching. It will elevate their self- esteem and teach them to meet your expectations. It was always exciting to see Dylan motivated to seek out wanted behaviors instead of those that were unwanted.

As mentioned earlier, one technique that we've used and found to be effective is ignoring unwanted behavior while *always* keeping an eye on him to make sure he was safe. We would avoid eye contact and not engage with him until he stopped the behavior. When he realized this we would offer praise.

Trust your judgement and follow through. Again, consistency, while sometimes difficult, is imperative. If you give in because you are stressed out in the moment, it will be confusing to your child and make it harder for them to correct unwanted behaviors.

For children who cannot read verbal cues or struggle with verbal communication it's important to remain neutral and calm. Pay attention to the tone and sound of your voice when speaking to your child. Notice how your child can recognize the differences (i.e. loud and soft noises result in different reactions).

Focus on the Positives

Using sticker charts are a simple, yet effective, form of positive reinforcement that can be extremely helpful in curbing behavioral issues associated with autism. Be sure to use your child's special interests as motivators. For example, Dylan loved the Thomas the Train show, the train store, train shows and train rides, so we were always looking for fun train stickers online (we also took him to train events that he would enjoy and used these moments to teach and motivate him). Customize the sticker chart for your child and make it as simple or complicated as you want. Provide a sticker for each day he/she behaves well. When Dylan reached a pre-determined number of stickers, he earned the item or trip to the park or train store. Choose rewards that will motivate your child and that you can deliver consistently, for example, additional play time, more time on the iPad, going to the park, etc. Our ABA therapist discouraged us from using candy or sweets, new toys or give monetary rewards because they would be difficult to maintain long term. Praise your child often, as this will keep them motivated, and never take away stickers as a consequence for an unwanted behavior, as this is something he/she worked hard for. If he/she didn't earn a sticker, review the goals on the behavior chart, focus on the positives and be encouraging for long-term success. Avoid reprimanding your child for not earning a sticker.

Consequences

Consequences teach accountability, responsibility and problem-solving at all ages. It's important to use this approach effectively and properly by not criticizing your child. The goal is to provide learning opportunities and raise their self-esteem.

We learned a lot about consequences from Brendan during our daily ABA sessions. He explained that there are two types of consequences: natural and logical. *Natural consequences* are the inevitable result of a child's actions. For example, Dad urges child to put on his coat, child goes outside to play in the cold without wearing a coat. The natural result is the child gets cold. The result is a consequence of a choice the child made. When this occurs, offer empathy and help the child reflect on and learn new strategies. *Logical consequences* happen as a result of a child's actions/choices, but are imposed by the parent/caregiver. For example, the child rides their bike into the road after he/she was told not to. The logical consequence would be for the mother to take away the bike while they are playing. Logical consequences are effective when a child's actions could affect their safety. They must be related to the behavior, respectful, reasonable, and delivered with empathy.

While both natural and logical consequences are effective, there is an important difference. Natural consequences don't always occur as a result of poor behaviors, but logical consequences, which correlate directly to your child's behavior, can help him/her clearly understand and implement changes.

It is not easy to raise a child on the spectrum (or any child, for that matter) but their behavior, over time, can be managed effectively with gentle positive techniques. Physical discipline should be avoided. It only teaches the child that hitting is an acceptable response to a negative situation. Providing praise, implementing calming techniques and constant redirection will put your child on the right path to better behavior.

Tips to Help Parents Discipline a Child
who has Special Needs

- Be Consistent

- Learn About Your Child's Diagnosis

- Define Expectations

- Reward Good Behavior

- Use Consequences

- Use Clear + Simple Messages

- Establish a Routine

- Believe in Your Child

- Listen to Your Child

- See the Suggestions on page 95 for helping your child balance their emotions and stay grounded.

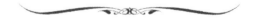

Journal the strategies or plan you have in place.

Are they effective for your child?

_____
_____
_____
_____
_____
_____
_____
_____
_____
_____
_____

Is there something you'd like to implement?

_____
_____
_____
_____
_____
_____
_____
_____
_____
_____
_____

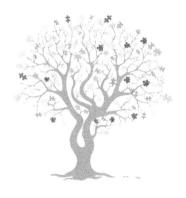

9

Change and Transition

"Once you choose hope,
anything is possible."
—Christopher Reeve

Knowing the difference between *change* and *transition* is important when determining how to best meet your child's needs. Change is an inevitable part of life; for example, being at home and starting nursery school, going from nursery to preschool, from preschool to elementary, and so on. Transitions are moving from one activity to another over the course of a day, and they are particularly difficult for individuals with ASD because they rely on structure and routine to navigate life. This was always our biggest issue with Dylan – asking him to stop one activity (that was highly preferred) and start another (possibly less preferred and something that he needed to do). Making this request often triggered behavior problems that resulted in a full blown meltdown. Dylan was often confused and overwhelmed by his emotions and it was up to me and Anthony to help him work through it. Staying calm was key.

Sometimes, transitions include change, like when one is meeting new people, attending family events, going to a new or different environment with new sights and sounds, or beginning new routines and activities. Transitions can be extremely stressful, no matter what age or how big or small the change may be. Now a teenager, Dylan still struggles with transitions; however, he no longer responds outwardly with tantrums or outbursts. Instead, he has had to learn internally how to cope and respond accordingly when he feels this way. Learning to manage these transitions early on has made a huge impact on his well-being and relationships with others.

Transition strategies are techniques used to support individuals with ASD during changes in or disruptions to activities, settings, or routines. Techniques can be used before a transition occurs, or during/after a transition. They can be presented verbally, auditory, or visually. Children with ASD often have a script in their mind for everything that happens throughout their day, so consider all the changes, prepare your child with a "head's up," and be supportive when they occur.

Below you'll find a "toolbox" of common strategies we've used over the years. They are the go-tos we discovered through trial and error, lots of worrying, planning, tears and, after working through a difficult time, joy.

Toolbox Strategies

– Create a calendar.

– Follow a schedule.

– Create social stories or photo books.

– Consider using a timer. Allow more time between activities and provide warnings for how long the child has left to participate in the activity.

– Make sure the child knows and understands what is coming next and give him or her something to look forward to.

– Don't forget a transition object. Let them bring a highly preferred toy, book, or other object. It can be designated for difficult times of day. Sometimes this is all it takes!

– Practice the art of distraction (i.e. singing)

– First, next, then, last

– Provide videos of new places, environments if possible.

– Provide calming strategies so your child knows where they can go to calm or access sensory tools.

– Use the art of distraction to help your child move from point A to point B with singing, dancing, bubbles, and toys.

– Create a consistent way of signaling that an activity is over (i.e. singing the clean-up song to put toys away).

– Practice makes perfect. Repeat practice trails and try new ideas!

– Don't rush things! Have fun and be patient. Structure and consistency are KEY. Prepare ahead of time.

Consider creating a calendar. Children with autism do not have the organizational or planning skills to navigate the day successfully. They do not inherently understand or follow routines and often experience stress and anxiety when they are unsure what to do. For parents, it's a constant balancing act to provide the structure they thrive in while teaching them about change.

A calendar helps your child know what is coming, what to plan for, and how to get organized. It also teaches your child the days of the week, months and year; it also creates excitement, for example, when counting down to birthdays, holidays or special events. Planning ahead can help with daily transitions and reduce anxiety. Start talking about the event that's coming, make a Social Story about the place and people and present it in a positive way to get positive results.

Following a schedule everyday has really helped our family, as everyone knows what to expect and anticipate. I've tried many ideas over the years (usually found on Pinterest) to create a family calendar, but I've found keeping it as simple as possible is the best way to stay on track. That said, keeping Dylan's schedule separate has proved helpful to him. When creating or adding to your calendar, be sure to include your child, as it's a great way to open a conversation. If your child cannot read, explore the option of picture schedules.

Plan ahead. Trying to "hurry up" a child on the spectrum can be difficult as they will become upset or anxious. Get organized when you need extra time so you're not scrambling to find things at the last minute. Life can get messy, and we can't control every circumstance, but planning ahead will reduce your child's frustration and anxiety, as well as your own.

Back when Dylan struggled immensely with transitions, Brendan suggested we start using a timer. He explained that Dylan didn't understand what phrases like "five more minutes" meant, but being able to see and hear the timer would allow him to go from one activity to the next with greater ease. Indeed, the timer quickly became our best friend. For example, leaving the playground was difficult because it was a highly preferred activity. My husband and I would say, "Ten more minutes," then we would set the timer at the five-minute and two-minute marks to let him know it was getting close. When it went off for the last time, he knew it was time to leave. Brendan also pointed out that having the timer let Dylan know it was time to go, rather than me or Anthony, reduced his aggression towards us during transitions. Like everything, it took practice and time, but yielded excellent results.

The speech therapist provided another very helpful tip: we should provide verbal prompts and talk through activities and transitions. For example, getting ready for school involved multiple steps (i.e. going to the bathroom, washing hands and face, getting dressed, brushing teeth, putting on shoes, and carrying his backpack and lunch box to the car). Verbal prompting along the way created a sense of ease through these transitions and taught responsibility.

First, Then, Next, Last

A first/then chart is an amazing tool to help correct behavioral issues. This is a visual representation of what you want your child to do now (FIRST) and what will come after (THEN). The idea is to make the first task less desirable and to follow it up with some sort of reward. This process teaches them about the sequencing of events and gives them a heads up about what to expect.

Start by introducing "first, next," then expand that to "first, then, next." If your child begins to grasp three-step directions, you can try adding a fourth step: "first, then, next, last." These steps require *time and patience.* Keep it simple, as saying too much will overwhelm him/her. For example:

"**First** we'll get our shoes on, **then** we'll get in the car."

"**First** school**, then** park."

"**First**, we'll get dressed, **next** we'll have breakfast, **then** we'll leave for school."

"**First** we'll wake up, **then** we'll go the bathroom, **next** we'll get dressed, **last** we'll eat breakfast."

Plan ahead. Mornings were usually the most difficult, so it was important to prepare the night before so I could be at my best. If I didn't I found myself unorganized and felt rushed, which wasn't helpful for Dylan. Kids on the spectrum need extra time to go from one activity to another and to process following directions and the steps involved. Try to avoid rushing. It's easier said than done some days, but it is attainable when you plan ahead. Try to remind yourself to be patient and prepared, as your child will sense when you're overwhelmed and likely struggle to follow directions and follow through with tasks. When this happened in our home, a full-blown (and avoidable) meltdown inevitably followed. Many times I had to remind myself to do better the next time. Life happens and we need to allow ourselves some grace.

Positive reinforcement, praise and encouragement are needed and make a difference!

Even the simplest achievements build confidence and self-esteem, so recognize them and celebrate!

By acknowledging their success, they are learning to follow directions and get that "feel good" feeling that you're *proud* of them!

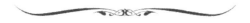

Journal about your toolbox of strategies.

Do you need to change things up?

_____

_____

_____

_____

_____

_____

_____

_____

_____

_____

_____

_____

_____

_____

_____

_____

_____

_____

_____

_____

_____

_____

_____

_____

_____

_____

_____

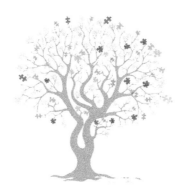

10

Sensory Playroom

"PLAY is the work of childhood."

—Mr. Rogers

One of my first jobs out of college was working as a recreational therapist in an assisted living setting. I loved it! My calendar focussed on art and music programs and I thouroughly enjoyed seeing the residents respond so positively. I learned to start meeting people where they were, through communication and activites that spoke to their values, needs, and emotions. I believe that once I understood this idea as a young professional, my vocation of serving others transformed and shifted my thoughts of how I wanted to be as a mother. In truth, I hadn't always planned on being a wife and mother; my focus was on my career. But God had other plans for me.

Not only am I a wife and mother (and love it), but a mother of a son with special needs. It's true that God doesn't give you more than you can handle; He knew I needed Dylan exactly the way he is to teach and help me grow as a person. I've always loved implementing music, play therapy and fun into Dylan's daily schedule, just as I did when I worked in assisted living. If you are interested in creating additional fun ways into your child's day, my suggestion is to meet with an Occupational Therapist to arrange a plan and suggestions to meet your child's needs. Another suggestion is to go to Pinterest and search keywords. For example: music + autism at home, autism + play at home, sensory play at home, and so on. You will find so many great, inexpensive or DIY exciting ideas!

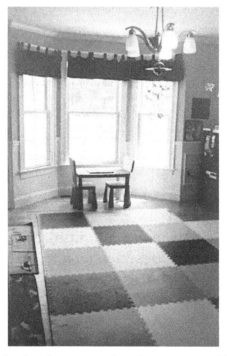

(Dylan's playroom when he was a toddler)

My husband and I turned our dining room into a playroom/ therapy room when Dylan was a toddler. It was just off the kitchen and made it easier to keep him safe and in one area when I had to put the wash in the dryer or do other housework. We spent hours in the playroom, and playing music kept it happy and upbeat. Other days, we'd play Disney movies for softer background noise. I'd go to the Dollar Store and purchase items from the teachers section (ABC posters, seasonal décor, counting posters) for the walls. It made the room bright, cherry and welcoming. Dylan and I became interested in art therapy together. With the music on, it calmed him and he would sit at the table with crayons and paper and scribble. Most of the time I hadn't a clue what it was, but I didn't care. I was happy that he was calm and engaged. I would put a string from one side of the wall to the other and hang his work each time he did something. He would point and smile at his work. I found that it boosted his self esteem. I would talk to him about what he created and teach him colors by pointing at what crayons he used.

What is Play and why is it so important?

Play is the work of children. It consists of those activities performed for self-amusement that have behavioral, social, and psychomotor rewards. It is child-directed and the rewards come from within the individual child. Our goal as parents is to make it enjoyable, spontaneous and use it to create memories.

Play and Autism

There are Social Stages of Play; however for children with ASD play is often solitary. Several factors contribute to the lack of social play. As we know, individuals with autism have communication deficits. They may not understand the language or social cues of peers, or have the ability to express their feelings effectively with others. Fortunately, play comes in many forms. The options are endless!

Do you remember that feeling as a child where you felt the excitement and happiness of play? Now is your chance to experience that with your child. Yes, cutting out specific time to allow yourself to be in that headspace may take practice, but the bond you will forge with your child is priceless.

Here are a few ideas to engage your child in active play ...

- Try to incorporate "favorites" or "highly preferred toys" to get their attention
- Add in new ideas and toys slowly by making the "unknown" more familiar.
- Celebrate small and large successes; build on those moments.
- Be resourceful by talking to others for ideas and research. My go-to is Pinterest.
- Don't give up if you don't succeed at first!
- Be patient. You've got this!

I've included some suggestions that you may want to include in your play/sensory room at home. We tried many of these items in the earlier years. I would borrow from mothers I had met at EI playgroups or buy them secondhand in case he didn't do well with it. If you don't have access to these suggestions, you can modify and use what you have. Get creative!

Suspended equipment. Swings are a sensory favorite for a good reason. They not only offer vestibular input and proprioceptive input, they are FUN! Swings at the playground or in your backyard are great, but so are indoor swings, so long as you have the right structures and hookups. Depending on your space, you might be able to install suspended equipment in a ceiling joist; you'll also need to be sure you make space for a stand or swing frame. We found ours at IKEA. A child's day can completely turn around after getting some much-needed sensory input.

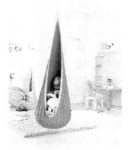

Balance and sensory tools. A balance beam is a wonderful basic piece of equipment for any sensory room. Balance boards, steppingstones, and E-Z steppers are great alternatives that are space savers and portable. Balance beams offer vestibular input for children with gravitational insecurity.

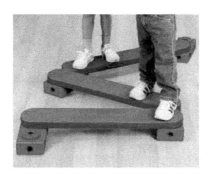

Tactile media. A low table and a shallow storage container can serve as a sensory bin anytime. A sand/water table is great for flexibility and ease of use/clean up. Rice, beans, kinetic sand, pasta, and shaving cream are fun tactile media to explore. Putty and Play-Doh are go-tos to help develop hand muscles and fine motor skills. Another fun idea is using shaving cream art for sensory play ..Pinterest it!

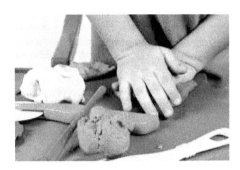

Trampoline. Whether you're outdoors or indoors, jumping on a trampoline delivers proprioceptive and vestibular input to people of all ages. Trampolines come in several different shapes and sizes; some versions have a handle for younger children and others can accommodate several users at once. There are options available for smaller spaces too.

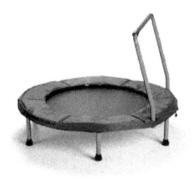

Crash mat. Fun DIY project! A cushion filled with foam ends, balls, or even air make a great landing space. Kids can drag them around, toss them, climb under or flop onto them.

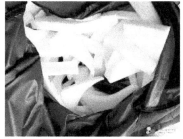 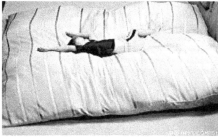

Climbing and Go Vertical! Climbing has many benefits, including strengthening, coordination and motor planning. It's an awesome way to help develop cognitive skills and problem-solving skills. There are temporary and removable options if you have the space; these can also be paired with suspended equipment and doorway swing hookups. Other options include nets, ropes and ladders that can be interchanged to offer different experiences and levels of challenges. Just Google "doorway swing" to see what's available. Climbing is a great example of vestibular and proprioceptive combination. It tests balance while pulling and stepping provides heavy work to those joints. Best of all, climbing is FUN and EXCITING!

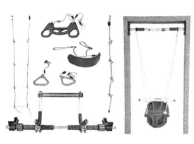 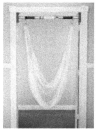 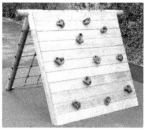

Body Sock. This FUN sensory-based tool is used to provide proprioceptive input and is flexible and creative for play. Body socks are stretchy pieces of Lycra that your child can get completely inside, curl up in a ball or stretch out (there is an opening for the head). They are portable, flexible, and a great option for children who struggle with sensory regulation.

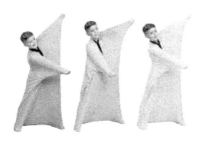

Ball. A yoga ball, stability ball or physio ball is a flexible tool for a sensory space. Using a small ball as a seat allows for some movement to help promote focus and attention. With an adult, a larger ball can be rolled over to target upper body strength, sat on to challenge postural control, used for deep pressure input as a "steam roller" or bounced on for vestibular input. Your child can use it by him or herself, getting sensory input by rolling it up the wall, dribbling it, bouncing on it, or kicking it against the wall.

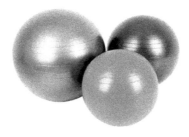

Kids with autism who spin or bounce are usually trying to stimulate their **vestibular system**, or inner ear. The inner ear helps with balance, and it also helps the body know when it is moving and how fast it is moving.

Tunnel. A fold-up or collapsible tunnel can encourage crawling or be used as an obstacle course. Kids can crawl through inside on their bellies, pull in a blanket or a pillow to decompress and relax. Dylan used to think he was hiding and no one could see him. It was fun!

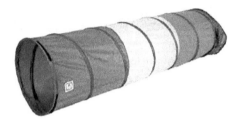

Vertical surfaces. The EI therapist suggested we purchase a paper roll to hang on the wall, a chalkboard or whiteboard to get him working in an upright vertical surface. Another option is using the surface as a creative felt board with a topic of their choice. This will promote and encourage visual motor skills by grasping the crayon or chalk. Another fun option would be to add a large piece of paper and finger paint.

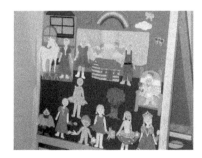

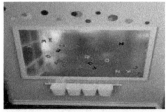

Super Easy DIY Magnet Board

Busy Boards DIY. My husband and I love DIY projects, and we made this one an adventure! We created ours by gathering items at the Dollar Store, Goodwill and our own garage and things around the house and adhering for safety. Here are a couple examples.

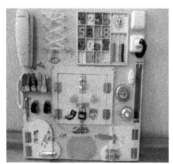 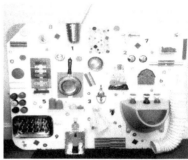

Additional ideas: Bean bags, hammock swing, swim noodles, orange cones, basketball hoop, beads, ball pit, hula hoops, gymnastic mat, hopscotch mat, pogo jumper, wobble chair, jump rope, and stretchy bands.

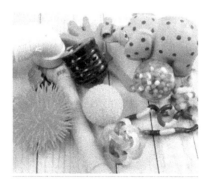

When you have a child with autism, sensory toys have the potential to be amazing and serve a double purpose. Finding toys that your child is interested in and provides the sensory input they crave can be challenging. On the other hand, there is no better feeling than finding the fun sensory toys that can help your child push past their fears and still have fun! It's a sense of accomplishment for both of you!

Fidget Toys...

are often used to provide sensory input in a less distracting way. They can help improve concentration and attention to tasks by allowing the brain to filter out the extra sensory information (e.g. listening to a lesson in the classroom, paying attention to a book during circle time).

Sensory Toys...

are specially designed to engage a child's attention, both cognitively and physically, by stimulating one or more of the five senses: sight, sound, touch, smell, and taste.

Sensory Tools...

include Thera-putty, Play Dough, moon sand, writing grips, hand-held stretchy items, drawing, and fidget tools. Areas of Learning Impacted include touch, tactile input, fine motor coordination, and hand strength.

Joint Compressions and the Wilbarger Brushing Protocol

When Dylan received EI services, my husband and I took a class on calming joint compressions, as recommended by the OT. We found that he responded well to it.

Throughout the class, we were taught about calming joint compressions and sensory brushing, both of which reset your child's sensory system. The goal is to help their overloaded sensory system stop, relax and then reboot itself. It provides better focus and it can lessen some of the stimuli going to the nervous system. The instructor explained that it can be thought of as hitting pause on an overactive system.

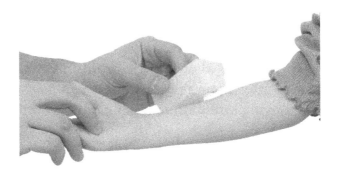

The Therapressure Brush is the sensory brush designed by Patricia Wilbarger, an occupational therapist who developed the Wilbarger Brushing Protocol (also known as "brushing"). It is the standard used for most occupational therapists. Some of the benefits of brushing include improved attention span, improved ability to transition between daily activities, a decreased fear or discomfort of being touched, enhanced coordination, and better self-regulation. The brushing technique is recommended every two hours while the child is awake. You may also want to have the brush available anytime your child needs that type of pressure.

At first, I spent some time observing the OT while she brushed Dylan's arms, legs and feet. When I noted that her hand never left his body, she explained that not breaking contact was key here.

Next comes the joint compressions (for best results, joint compressions *always* follow brushing.) You want to press on each joint three times in a row. For example, you grab the shoulder and the elbow and press at the same time. The same goes for hips, knees and the other joints. *Before trying joint compressions, please consult with your doctor and or physical therapist for instruction and safety purposes.*

Your child may only allow the brushing, but it's better than nothing. If compressions are not an option, you can try jumping jacks, sit-ups, or exercise they prefer. The goal is to get your child's body into sync *prior* to asking anything of him/her. Mornings are best, and our OT provided us with a chart to follow. We weren't perfect at the schedule (because life happens), but the most important thing was to be consistent. We also did it before heading off to a family gathering, birthday party, or other special event.

When the OT introduced these concepts to us, Anthony and I listened but were not really buying into the idea. As always, we asked her for further instruction, researched, and spoke with Dylan's doctor, but what sold us was the tremendous differences we saw they made for Dylan. It was so dramatic that afterward he was able to start and complete a task, sit long enough to color, focus to play, etc. In the event that you are running late or something has come up, consider using a weighted blanket or weighted vest while in route to wherever you're going. The idea is to help calm the sensory system when it's taxed or stressed. One year my husband and I wanted to attend a Christmas tree lighting. The OT helped us create a Sensory Backpack for Dylan to carry around. The weight gave him proprioceptive input and allowing him to feel "grounded." All of these ideas are part of a sensory diet that is imperative for a child on the spectrum's daily success.

An excellent resource around Joint Compressions is www. kidsplaysmarter.com, created by occupation therapist Amy Smith. There is a terrific article there in which Smith explains the concept of proprioceptive input. Proprioception refers to pressure on the body's joints, muscles, and bones that then elicit chemical, physiological, and physical changes in the body. Our bodies need proprioceptive input to improve our body awareness, body organization, postural security; and once the body becomes more secure and organized it can then relax, calm down, and handle stress in a more efficient manner. Joint compressions also utilize human touch which has been shown to facilitate the release of dopamine and norepinephrine. Dopamine and norepinephrine are two neurotransmitters that are responsible for mood regulation, motivation, lowering anxiety levels, and lowering depression. As Smith wrote, "So, by doing joint compressions with your child you are actually getting 'double the bang for your buck' as you are reaping the benefits of both proprioception and touch combined."

This will not only help your child on a physical and physiological level, but it will also help you and your child to bond as you complete this calming activity together.

Joint compressions are great to help calm your child and can be done multiple times a day if needed. Below are some suggested times to try this practice:

- Before entering a stressful environment such as school, sports, or work
- Before your child goes to bed
- Before your child needs to complete a task
- During a daily sensory diet or plan at home or school

- When your child is overly active and can't seem to sit still
- When your child is having difficulty focusing
- Proactively to maintain healthy behaviors, motivations, and attention span

Moreover, joint compressions also benefit children with ADD, ADHD, Sensory Processing Disorder, and anxiety, behavioral, or emotional difficulties

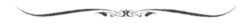

How do you connect and create memories with your child? Do you enjoy playing?

_____

_____

_____

_____

_____

_____

_____

_____

_____

_____

_____

What are some activities you'd like to try with your child?

_____

_____

_____

_____

_____

_____

_____

_____

_____

_____

_____

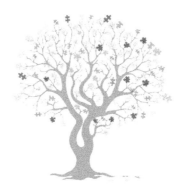

11

You Matter Too...

"Keep taking time for yourself until you're you again."
— Lalah Delia

Find Your Village

Surround yourself with people who will understand and take the time to listen and hear your thoughts, fears and positive strides. When we become parents, no one hands us a manual for what is right, wrong or what to do next.

I want you to know that *you are not alone*. The autism community is strong, supportive and available to help each other along the way.

Look for the helpers when you need them, for they are around you and want to help. Find ways to tap into parent groups and support groups. Find the confidence to put yourself out there to participate in play dates and groups and educate others around you so they understand your journey.

I know that it's hard some days. I know the raw feelings of being emotionally and physically drained and unsure of where to turn and whether you're doing the right or wrong thing for your child. I know that overwhelming feeling, that scared feeling, that feeling that others are judging you and your family or your child. You just keep doing what you know and believe is right for your child.

I have met families that reside in cities and have services available right at their fingertips and I have met families that live in more rural areas with the most limited services available. You have to work with your present circumstances in order to work for a better trajectory for your child. If you live in a rural area that doesn't have services available to come to your home, reach out to the closest Autism Society for suggestions and support; watch podcasts and free online educational videos on specific topics. Keep filling your "toolbox" for resources when you need them.

Thankfully, resources are just a google search away. Pinterest can offer a wealth of information and free charts as well. I have enclosed charts in this book and they will be available to you to print PDFs for free on the website *PuttingThePiecesTogetherBook.com*

Autism Parents

Most autism parents I've met are fearless, passionate and a force to be reckoned with, who will endlessly advocate and protect their child. You often hear them called "Warrior Moms and Dads." We fight for services, healthcare decisions and our children's rights to receive an appropriate education. We research the facts, seek out treatment and share stories to help others. Our relentless love and devotion to our children and families is not taken lightly. It's what we know and what we do.

Dylan's autism diagnosis broke me down to my very core, drastically changed life as I knew it and brought up thoughts and feelings I had never experienced or even knew existed. At the same time, autism has nurtured and soothed my soul. I always had this inner tug at my heart, reminding me that I was willing to do whatever I could to help Dylan be the best version of himself. I had to be doctor, teacher, therapist, lawyer and CEO, all at the same time; more importantly, I had to learn to rely on my intuition to make quick important decisions. I quickly learned that I can be and do all these things when I need to, but I am always his mom first.

Self-Care and Self-Love

Choose to love yourself a little bit more. If you find a five-minute hair and makeup routine that makes you feel good and confident to take on your day, go for it! If it's exercise, doing yardwork, meeting up with a friend for coffee, or just getting time to yourself to read – do it, whatever it is that "fills your bucket." Your child deserves a confident, happy parent and most importantly, you deserve to feel good about yourself.

Years ago, I read a quote that both caused my heart to sink and sparked something within me: "You were someone before you were a mom and she still matters." Prior to being a mom I had been someone different, with very different dreams and goals. I made time for myself. I used to have girls' nights, sing karaoke, or go shopping with a friend.

Then motherhood came in and it was all-consuming, and I mean *all-consuming*. As a new mother of a child with special needs, I now felt guilty making time for myself because Dylan's needs mattered more, or so I thought. I admired my friends and other moms who prioritized themselves. I struggled with that during the earlier years. I never put myself on the calendar. I had to crash and burn and learn the hard way. I know from experience that it's important to prioritize you too. Don't hold off. I went years losing myself, forgetting what made me happy and filling my own bucket because I was so busy filling up others,' and I can tell you it's hard to come back from there.

Rock bottom came ten years ago when I was diagnosed with an autoimmune disease. The symptoms come in waves and of course stress is one of the biggest triggers. I was forced to learn how to care for myself emotionally and keep it in check so I could physically be well. If I wasn't at my best due to autoimmune issues, it would make for a harder day, that's for sure. My husband has been my rock and has the ability to know when I'm taxed out and need more support. Over the years, through finding the right doctor and chiropractor, vitamin therapy and holistic practices, I am in remission with occasional flares. You can bet I've learned to take time for the things I now enjoy and find balance.

Today, I have come full circle. I know what is important and who is important – who I'm willing to invest my limited amount of energy into. I can no longer keep friends or family in my life who cannot respect that or meet me there. That's what this journey has taught me over the years. It has taken me a long time, but I've become comfortable with who I am now. I like the new me.

Finding My Voice

In the early days, one of the hardest things to deal with were the reactions of others when Dylan had a meltdown in public. It took all I had somedays to keep it together, and their stares and comments were enough to put me over the edge. I wanted to be the mom who could make a difference and speak out on behalf of my child, but I felt too overwhelmed and insecure to do so.

One day, I decided to break down those barriers in my mind and to put a voice to what I was experiencing. I went to see a counselor who was well-versed in the needs of ASD to process what I was feeling and learn to respond constructively to the stares and comments. Going to the counselor helped me to grow as a person, wife and mother. I eventually invited Anthony to join in a few sessions as well. She helped us navigate difficult situations while staying connected. Her professionalism validated our parenting efforts and strengthened us as a couple when it was needed most. She provided us with the tools we needed and explained that our child's autism diagnosis would not ruin our relationship, how we responded to it might.

Learning to work through my feelings allowed me to finally feel calm and re-discover the gal I used to be. In continually educating myself, I was also preparing to educate others. I was evolving into a confident mother who was accepting of this journey and felt empowered when I needed to. If you are struggling with this or something similar, I encourage you to seek out a counselor to find your voice too.

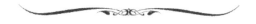

How do you fill your bucket to practice self-care to care for YOU?

_____

_____

_____

_____

_____

_____

_____

_____

_____

_____

Do you reach out when you need help or a break?
Make a list of what you need in your
life to find that balance.

_____

_____

_____

_____

_____

_____

_____

_____

_____

_____

_____

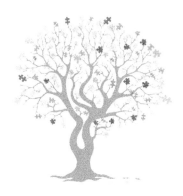

12

Let's Wrap This Up!

"Autism doesn't come with a manual.
It comes with a parent who never gives up."

—Kerry Magro

Finding Joy in Your Journey

Listen to your child's needs, you know them best. Continue celebrating the unique challenges of parenting them. There will always be charts and statistics, but you know what your child is capable of. Dylan has surpassed each goal because we refused to give up, no matter how difficult things got. Your strength will come when you need it most, especially on the hardest days. And when the hard days get to be too much, look back and see how far you've come. You will be so proud of yourself, your child and the progress you've made as a family. Each day our children are learning, changing and growing before our eyes. If they can't do something today doesn't mean it's not going to happen, they just may need more time. You are your child's voice and advocate. Your child needs you to believe in them and in yourself.

As special needs parents we often become overwhelmed by all the things our children need to learn. We are often reminded what developmental milestones are coming and what they "should" be doing according to the professionals. If you've ever thought, *Should I be doing more, teaching more? Is there something I've missed?*, you're not alone. I think we've all had that feeling at one time or another. Stay in your own lane, and continue discovering the unique beauty of your child. Remember and celebrate the growth they've experienced – the hours, months, days, and years of practice and hard work. Remember the emotions, the tears and the patience required of us each day. Somedays you may feel like giving up but, please, keep going! You've got this! Continue being resourceful, learning and educating yourself. Read, join, talk, get involved and be your child's advocate.

For me and Anthony, parenting has involved a lot of trial and error, asking a lot of questions and doing a lot of research. We've kept the lines of communication open, talking about things, the ways he has grown and changed. The word "toolbox" is still part of our daily vocabulary. When Dylan was in EI and preschool, our "toolbox" was always full. We had multiple therapists offering valuable information and doctors' input and suggestions. Over the years, however, information is not quite as easy to come by, and our "toolbox" is often low on resources and sometimes even empty. There are days we aren't sure what to do or how to handle situations that come up for our teenage son, but we figure it out.

We hope our story can help others by becoming more knowledgeable through our experiences. Autism has strengthened us as a family unit. It has also nurtured and softened my soul in ways that are innumerable and indescribable. I wish you and your family a wonderful journey filled with hope, joyful memories, lots of love, and success. Most of all, I hope I have encouraged you to "keep on keeping on – you've got this!"

Xo,

K

Resources

What is Applied Behavior Analysis? Retrieved from https://www.autismspeaks.org/applied-behavior-analysis-aba-0

Greenspan, Stanley, MD & Wieder, Serena, PhD. *DIR™ Floortime Model.* Retrieved from https://www.stanleygreenspan.com/swf/The%20DIR%20Floor-time%20Model.pdf

Barbera, Dr. Mary Lynch, *The Verbal Behavior Approach: How to Teach Children with Autism and Related Disorders.* Jessica Kingsley Publishing. 2007

What is PECS? Retrieved from https://pecsusa.com/pecs/

Smith, Amy, OTR/L, MA; Occupational Therapist, "Joint Compressions for Calming." Retrieved from https://kidsplaysmarter.com/joint-compressions-calming/

Wilbarger, P., & Wilbarger, J. L. (1991). *Sensory defensiveness in children aged 2-12: An intervention guide for parents and other caretakers.* Santa Barbara, Calif: Avanti Educational Programs.

About the Author

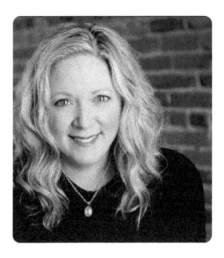

Kimberly Caggiano lives in a small town in the South with her loving husband Anthony and their two amazing boys. In her free time when she is not busy with her family, she enjoys design, decorating and painting furniture.

CPSIA information can be obtained
at www.ICGtesting.com
Printed in the USA
JSHW051507140920
7747JS00005B/8